'This book had a powerful effect on my body, mind and heart. As I kept on reading it, each cell in my body was lighting up with warmth, joy and happiness. This delightful book will transform millions of lives.'

GOSIA GORNA, AUTHOR OF THE EXPANSION GAME

'Dr David Hamilton possesses the rare talent of being able to make complex science easy for anyone to understand. Using leading-edge scientific research, which he brings to life with personal stories, he teaches us how acts of kindness, either given or received, have a direct effect that is measurable and capable of influencing our health, our happiness, our relationships and even how fast we age. In the context of today's global culture this is a much-needed, brilliant, unique and potentially life-changing read. Using Kindness as the alchemist, everyone can glean a nugget of gold from this book.'

DR ANN HUTCHISON, BVMS MRCVS

'This is a rare book. I've spent 20 years trying to connect the "individual" with the "company". I have tried every talent management technique under the sun. The Five Side Effects of Kindness connects the dots. If you place kindness and compassion as the heart of what you do, you will create a ripple effect that will benefit the "individual" and the "company" in equal measure. This is a book you can use to embrace, as David calls it, "the spirit of kindness", a scientifically proven phenomenon that can make a real difference to your health and happiness, and to those who are touched by such kindness. It is a truly inspirational and uplifting book. I thoroughly recommend it at all levels.'

GLEN HALL, CEO OF GOSFORTH 22 AND AUTHOR OF THE LAST DRUID

*'David Hamilton is not only a man with a vision for all mankind, but uniquely has the scientific background to deliver his message with great credibility and lucidity. When this is combined with the expression of his deep sense of humility and humanity, as in this book, we have the gift of further enlightenment to help us move forward with a renewed sense of courage, caring, commitment and hope.'*

DREW PRYDE, CHAIRMAN OF THE SCOTTISH INSTITUTE
OF BUSINESS LEADERS (SIBL CIC)

# THE FIVE
# SIDE EFFECTS OF
# KINDNESS

# THE FIVE
# SIDE EFFECTS OF
# KINDNESS

## This Book Will Make You Feel Better,
## Be Happier & Live Longer

### DAVID R. HAMILTON PhD

**HAY HOUSE**

Carlsbad, California • New York City • London
Sydney •Johannesburg • Vancouver • New Delhi

First published and distributed in the United Kingdom by:
Hay House UK Ltd, Astley House, 33 Notting Hill Gate, London W11 3JQ
Tel: +44 (0)20 3675 2450; Fax: +44 (0)20 3675 2451; www.hayhouse.co.uk

Published and distributed in the United States of America by:
Hay House Inc., PO Box 5100, Carlsbad, CA 92018-5100
Tel: (1) 760 431 7695 or (800) 654 5126
Fax: (1) 760 431 6948 or (800) 650 5115; www.hayhouse.com

Published and distributed in Australia by:
Hay House Australia Ltd, 18/36 Ralph St, Alexandria NSW 2015
Tel: (61) 2 9669 4299; Fax: (61) 2 9669 4144; www.hayhouse.com.au

Published and distributed in the Republic of South Africa by:
Hay House SA (Pty) Ltd, PO Box 990, Witkoppen 2068
Tel/Fax: (27) 11 467 8904; www.hayhouse.co.za

Published and distributed in India by:
Hay House Publishers India, Muskaan Complex, Plot No.3, B-2,
Vasant Kunj, New Delhi 110 070
Tel: (91) 11 4176 1620; Fax: (91) 11 4176 1630; www.hayhouse.co.in

Distributed in Canada by:
Raincoast Books, 2440 Viking Way, Richmond, B.C. V6V 1N2
Tel: (1) 604 448 7100; Fax: (1) 604 270 7161; www.raincoast.com

A catalogue record for this book is available from the British Library.

ISBN: 978-1-78180-813-9

Interior images: 48, 59, 69, 79, 89 © Beth Rivett-Carnac

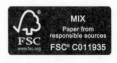

*In the sweetness of friendship, let there be laughter and sharing of pleasures. For in the dew of little things, the heart finds its morning and is refreshed.*

KAHLIL GIBRAN, THE PROPHET

# CONTENTS

# ACKNOWLEDGEMENTS

I am grateful to the following people for their invaluable contributions to this book:

Elizabeth Caproni, for her love and support throughout the writing process, for helpful suggestions and for patiently bearing with me during my sometimes long hours.

Lizzie Henry, my editor, for once again working magic in turning my draft into a finished article and ultimately making me look better as a writer.

Ann Hutchison and Joe Hayes, who read through the first draft and offered me invaluable feedback and insights that greatly enhanced the book.

All the staff of Hay House UK for all that they do to support me as an author.

The staff at Caffè Nero in Stirling, where I spent many mornings working on this book, for helping create an ideal atmosphere in which to work. And thanks to Caffè Nero as a company for creating such great-tasting coffee (and blueberry muffins).

Ems Harrington for supplying some stories for the book from her Facebook Group ('The Delight of Kindness') and for being the shining model of kindness that she is. And to all the people who shared stories of kindness, both those who made the book and the equally inspiring ones for whom I simply couldn't find room.

Bethany Rivett-Carnac for producing great illustrations that enhanced some of the specific points I was trying to make.

Robert Holden for his encouragement as I wrote this book and for being a sounding board when I needed one.

My mum, for teaching by example and showing me the power of kindness.

And last and certainly not least, my dog, Oscar, who passed away in November 2014, for helping me become the person I am now.

# INTRODUCTION

*Why Kindness is Good for You* was my fourth book, published in February 2010. About a year later, I wrote a blog for my website that was based on some of the content from the book, called 'The Five Side Effects of Kindness'.

As with all the blogs I write, I posted it and then left it alone. But a few years later, I started to check my web statistics – how many people visit my site every month, which pages are being viewed, etc. – and I noticed that whenever I posted a blog, the number of views would peak that day and gradually drop over the next few days. But that hadn't happened with 'The 5 Side Effects of Kindness'. It was still getting large numbers of views. In fact, in many of the months since I'd posted it, it had had more views than when I'd first posted it. On average, it had been getting about 1,000 page views every month and over the five years it had become the most viewed blog on my website. It had been viewed in over 150 countries and people had even started making up little infographics with the side effects on them and posting them online.

So I decided to turn it into a book. There had been a lot more scientific research in the area of kindness since I'd first written *Why Kindness is Good for You*, so there was a wealth of new information to draw on. I took about 10 per cent of the content of *Why Kindness is Good for You*, rewrote it, restructured it, made it shorter and added 90 per cent new content. This is the result.

In this book, you'll learn how kindness alters the brain and how it dilates arteries and lowers blood pressure. You'll learn that it is an antidote to depression and that it slows the seven big processes of ageing and even ageing at the cellular level. And you'll learn that we're all wired for kindness. Despite what you might have been told, we're *not* inherently selfish. The truth is, we're inherently kind.

Someone asked me, 'Why "side effects"? Why not just "five benefits of kindness"?' The answer is that I feel that 'side effects' is a term more likely to capture people's attention. Also, we usually think of side effects in the context of the negative side effects of drugs. As a former scientist from the pharmaceutical industry, it feels good to be rebranding the term.

A side effect occurs along*side* what's intended. When we intend to be kind, we may not expect anything else to happen, but many things *do* happen.

So what are the five side effects of kindness? Well, I don't want to give too much away and deprive you of the fun of reading on, but in a nutshell, kindness makes us happier, it's good for the heart, it slows ageing, it improves our relationships and it's contagious. These are the five things that occur along*side* acts of kindness.

There's a chapter dedicated to each of these side effects in turn, in which you'll learn about how and why it happens, the science that proves it, how it plays out in our lives and how it affects children, adults and older people. Along the way, there are also a few stories of acts of kindness performed by ordinary people and 50 suggestions for acts of kindness you can do yourself.

As well as nuggets of wisdom and advice to enhance your life, there's even some relationship advice that's born out of research where scientists watched people interact for just 15 minutes and then predicted with over 90 per cent accuracy whether a relationship would stand the test of time or not. There are certain things that you can do that pretty much guarantee a relationship will last. And of course kindness is involved!

But before we dive into learning all about the five side effects of kindness, there are a few questions that often come up when I talk about the benefits of kindness. They are all along the lines of: 'Why should we be seeking to benefit from an act of kindness? Doesn't that make it selfish rather than kind?'

It's an important issue given that this book is about the benefits you get from being kind. Is kindness selfish if you know you'll benefit from it?

I've found the answer isn't quite 'yes' or 'no'. It really depends! What are you doing? Are you a) trying to benefit from being kind or b) aware that you benefit from kindness but being kind anyway because it's the right thing to do?

Most people assume that a) is selfish. Maybe! But I don't think we should be quite so black and white in our assessments of things. I think we would do well not to judge so much.

Before we jump to conclusions, let's look at a few scenarios. Being kind to people helps alleviate depression, so what if you are suffering from depression and decide to volunteer for a charity, knowing that it will help you feel better? Does that make you selfish or does it mean you're reaching out for help yourself?

What if, knowing that showing empathy is better for your heart than judging people, you choose to listen to someone? Is that choice a selfish one?

Or if, knowing that helping someone feels good and that connection warms the heart, you *refrain* from helping lest you taint the purity of your motives?

Not easy, is it?

Gratitude makes us happier too. Is it selfish, then, to count your blessings or to say 'thank you' because doing so will make you feel better?

The subject can become quite complex, but we can also make it astonishingly simple by just being kind anyway and leaving others to get on with things in their own way. That's become my philosophy on it. I think we can get too bogged down with questioning whether we are being selfish or not and that the time we waste thinking about it is time we could use to help others.

My motive for writing this book is to create a dialogue about kindness, to consider it in ways we might not have thought of before. Talking about kindness motivates us to be kind. But there are times when the best thing isn't to talk at all but just to get on out there and be kind!

I remember that when my dog, Oscar, was alive, I was well aware that playing with a dog boosted levels of the hormone oxytocin and that it was very good for the heart. Did I play with him more because I knew that? Was that on my mind when he brought a ball to me and nudged me as if to say 'Dad, come play with me'? What do you think?

In the moment of being kind, something takes over. We act kindly because something inside us knows it's the right thing to do. Any thoughts about benefits, or other reasons, just disappear and are replaced by a feeling of connection, a sense of compassion, a desire to see relief or a smile appear on a person's face (or a dog's tail start to wag) and a wish to know that the person we're helping will be okay.

Kindness is much bigger than any words and questions we can put around it. It's much bigger than our philosophies, than our debates about whether we're really altruistic or selfish. Kindness isn't black and white – it's multi-coloured.

In fact, kindness just *is*. It has its own spirit of sorts. We tap into this spirit the moment we help someone, whether it's holding a door open, saying, 'Thanks, I appreciate you,' buying a gift that we think someone will like or sharing someone's workload to help ease their stress.

Some say that kindness is a form of self-preservation. In a way, it is – it builds relationships and thus strengthens society. So, by extension, it ensures our protection and survival. But that's not just protection and survival of the individual, but of the whole.

I think our world – from the personal worlds of our households, places of work and communities to the wider world – always benefits from kindness.

Several years ago, while experiencing my mum's helping hand and witnessing the kindness she showed to everyone in the family, I realized that kindness brought people together.

The American cultural anthropologist Margaret Mead once said, 'Never doubt that a small group of thoughtful, committed citizens can change the world; indeed, it's the only thing that ever has.'

Inspired by these words, I formed my guiding philosophy: that a small group of people with compassion and kindness in their hearts could change the world.

In this modern interconnected world, there are no isolated acts of kindness. Kindness creates ripples in the fabric of human relationships and human society. These ripples impact the hearts and minds of other people, who in turn create ripples of their own. Each seemingly isolated act of kindness matters more than we think.

The Buddha once said, 'Thousands of candles can be lit from a single candle, and the life of the candle will not be shortened. Happiness never decreases by being shared.'

It's the same with kindness. The notion of giving suggests that we now have less. But with kindness we don't have less when we give, we have more. It's the 'kindness paradox'.

We are lifted by the spirit of kindness, too – when giving doesn't cause any stress, that is. But what if it does?

'It really bugs me when they don't say thanks.'

'They never do anything for me.'

These are very typical sentiments. There are two things to consider here.

First, we shouldn't wear ourselves out by giving and giving and giving, only for our kindness to be met with expectation or, worse, ingratitude. Everyone deserves to be appreciated. We might quite rightly wonder if there are other people, in other places, who might appreciate us more, because we have a right to that appreciation.

The other thing to consider at such times is that kindness is less stressful when there are no strings attached. Stress occurs when we expect something in return and don't get it. But it doesn't if we have no expectations, if we decide that 'This is who I am: I am kind' and leave it at that.

These two considerations are irrelevant for some people, because they have grateful people around them and people who show them kindness, but they are very relevant to those whose immediate family members, friends, colleagues, etc., just keep taking, without any appreciation whatsoever.

We each need to find our own balance point so that our needs are met, and this really depends on the context of our own lives – the people around us, our environment, what we do, where we work, our mental and emotional health, and our physical health. And if we are overstretched and underappreciated, we have to decide if we are happy to accept more of the same or if it's time for a change. We need to be kind to *ourselves*.

The world isn't a place where everyone is happy, where everyone has their needs met on a daily basis. So we need kindness. We need to show kindness to ourselves and others. We depend upon each other. Kindness holds the fabric of human society together.

I grew up in a small community in central Scotland. Everyone helped each other. Everyone looked out for each other. It wasn't uncommon to have a neighbour knock on our door and ask to borrow a cup of sugar, a few slices of bread or some milk. It was this sharing that knitted our community together.

Kindness benefits us all. That's an unavoidable fact. It makes us happier. That's an immediate gain. It's also good for the heart and it improves our relationships. If we live a lifetime of kindness, thousands of people might benefit from it and our lifetime will not be shortened by it. In fact, it will be extended.

My advice is to be kind because it's the right thing to do, because someone you know is suffering and needs help, because a random opportunity presents itself as you go about your day, because it's nice and because there's something in human nature that enjoys the connections we create through helping each other.

So let's just get on with being kind and enjoying the side effects.

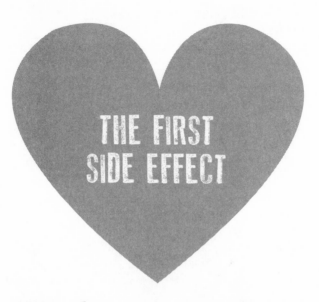

THE FIRST
SIDE EFFECT

# Kindness Makes Us Happier

*How beautiful a day can be*
*when kindness touches it.*
GEORGE ELLISTON

**Kindness [kahynd-nis]:** The quality of being friendly, generous and considerate.

**Other meanings:** Sympathy, gentleness, kind-heartedness, affection, benevolence, thoughtfulness, humanity, consideration, helpfulness, charity, human goodness, caring, compassion, goodwill, generosity, charitableness, a good turn.

**Kindnesses (plural):** More than one act of kindness.

*When I was getting off the train in Edinburgh, there was a young woman struggling to take two big, heavy suitcases and a big bag off the train. I took one of the cases off the train for her and then told her I would walk her to her next platform with the case. When we got there it was down loads of stairs (and the case weighed a ton), so the guy working at the station took it down the steps for me.*

*The woman was so grateful and kept saying how kind everyone was, as if she was surprised to see kindness, so*

*I was personally happy that she was having a really good experience with strangers!*

*I helped her onto the train and she gave me a big, huge hug and kept saying, 'God bless you!'*

*I was super touched by that. Two strangers on an empty train, hugging each other and not able to stop smiling. For me, there's no better high than helping someone.*

*I came away from that the lucky one!*

Eᴍs

'Why can't they just wait like everyone else?!' I'd yell as yet another car drove up the inside lane and slipped in front of me.

I'd get so furious. It was always at the same bit of road. Every time I was at the front of the queue and I suspected that this was what a car in the next lane was going to do, I'd have my foot poised, ready to slam it down on the accelerator so that I'd beat them to it and 'teach them a lesson'.

'Ha! That showed them!' I'd proclaim, with my heart racing and my eyes popping out of my head.

However, one day, as I was sitting in the queue with two cars in front of me, there was a car in the next lane with the indicator on in the hope that someone would let it in. As *the lights turned green, the two cars in front of me sped off, intentionally not letting it in.*

*But just as I was about to do the same, my foot eased off the accelerator. I realized that I didn't want to be stressed. I was tired of it. I was calm that day and I wanted to stay that way. I didn't want my blood pressure to be raised and my anger levels to be at a peak. So I gestured to the driver to say that it was okay and he went in front of me.*

*And you know what? I felt good – right away! It was much better than feeling as though my temples were going to pop from exasperation.*

*Then the guy flashed his hazard lights as a thank-you. This made me feel even more brilliant!*

*Since then I've let everyone go in front of me at that roundabout. It's no big deal in the grand scheme of things and I feel a zillion times better.*

ELISA

Most of us can probably recognize ourselves in these stories. Anger makes us stressed. Kindness, on the other hand, makes us feel good.

## Get Rich Quick

One of the wisest things my partner, Elizabeth, has ever said to me is: 'Being kind will make you rich – in happiness.'

It's true!

It's a side effect.

And the feelings that rise up inside us when we witness kindness or some other act of moral beauty, or when we give or receive kindness, lead to a whole array of positive health benefits. More on those later. For now, let's focus on how and why kindness makes us happier.

That kindness does make us happier is the everyday experience of people like you and me, but it's also the conclusion of a very large body of scientific research.

In a study led by Sonja Lyubomirsky, a psychology professor at the University of California, Riverside, for example, volunteers were asked to perform five acts of kindness per week for six weeks. They were compared to a control group, which was simply a group of people not intentionally being kind.

The many different acts of kindness the volunteers reported included donating blood, paying for someone's parking by filling the meter, helping a friend with homework, visiting an elderly relative and writing a thank-you letter.

Lyubomirsky found that the people who performed the acts of kindness became happier. Those who didn't, well, didn't. And it turned out that the greatest gains in happiness were when the five acts were done on the same day.[1]

# ACT OF KINDNESS

*Offer to carry an elderly person's shopping.*

In a different six-week study, nearly 500 people were divided into four groups. Two of the groups were asked to perform acts of kindness – one group for others and the other for the world (e.g. they might pick up litter). A third group was asked to do kind things for themselves (e.g. giving themselves a treat). The fourth group didn't perform any acts of kindness at all, for comparison purposes.

Each person had their psychological and emotional wellbeing measured before the study and after the six weeks.

After the six weeks, those who had been kind towards others and the world were happier. On the other hand, those who had been kind to themselves didn't report any significant change in happiness, which might come as a bit of a surprise to some.[2]

A similar study found that people who, in response to general questions covering different scenarios, listed things like 'volunteered my time', 'gave money to a person in need' or 'listened carefully to another's point of view' were happier, more satisfied with their lives and had a greater sense of wellbeing compared with people who were more self-focused.[3]

And when scientists at the University of British Columbia in Canada asked 632 people to make a daily record of how they spent their money over a period of a month, noting everything from paying bills to shopping, eating lunch and giving donations to charities and gifts to others, they found that the happiest people were those who listed spending money on others.

In another part of the same study, volunteers were given $5 or $20. Half were asked to spend the money on others by the end of the day and the other half were asked to spend it on themselves. At the end of the day, regardless of how much they'd been given, those who spent the money on others were happiest.[4]

It's quite natural, if we're feeling blue, to focus on ourselves and perhaps even treat ourselves in the hope that it will make us feel better. While it often does, and can be important for building self-esteem, these pieces of research show that a better option might actually be to help others or to make a difference to the world.

## ACT OF KINDNESS

*Allow someone in front of you
in the supermarket queue.*

This brings us back to the moral issue I discussed in the introduction. Is it wrong to be helpful if part of your reason for doing so is to feel better?

I would say that if someone benefits from your help, then it's not wrong. Part of your reason for helping is that you're reaching out because you need help too, so you're *helping each other*.

When we help others, it's sometimes the connection we crave, and it's the connection that creates happiness.

Some of the greatest pleasure I ever experienced was in helping Oscar. He was a yellow Labrador, full of life and happiness. He passed away in November 2014 at the age of two. He had bone cancer and we did everything we could to help him. It's hard to put into words the sense of connection and happiness – yes, happiness, even though we feared he was dying – that came from giving him what he wanted, what made him happy: toys, food, walks, play. When he smiled – yes, he smiled (a lot) – and wagged his tail ferociously, our hearts simply filled up.

Showing him love, kindness and affection every day brought me out of the fear of losing him. It was a difficult time, but the happiness I received from loving him was a reward that is etched in my heart and is a treat I still get to enjoy every time I think of him.

## Kindness to Ourselves

In some of the studies above, kindness only made people happier when they were kind to others and not themselves, or when they gave money away instead of spending it on themselves. This shouldn't be taken to mean that treating ourselves *can't* make us feel better.

My experience is that treating ourselves does in fact make us happier in the short term, but only when we do it as a statement of self-love. It has to be a statement that our own needs matter. It's especially powerful when we've been neglecting our needs for some time.

That's what I learned from workshop participants after I wrote my latest book, *I Heart Me: The Science of Self-Love*. Participants who treated themselves on purpose, as a declaration that they mattered or they were good enough, reported feeling happier and raising their self-esteem.

It's popular to think that being kind to ourselves is selfish, that we're placing our own needs ahead of someone else's. But it's not quite so black and white.

Being kind to ourselves is much more than just buying ourselves presents or treating ourselves in some other way. Kindness to ourselves can be declaring that we've had enough of a certain set of circumstances and determining to change things. It can be acknowledging that we deserve something better and we value ourselves enough to do something about it.

Kindness to ourselves is also shown in standing up for ourselves, in deciding that we deserve to be treated with kindness and respect. It can be shown, too, in the decision to be ourselves and not the person everyone expects us to be.

These ways of being kind to ourselves do make us happier, in my experience. They produce a sense of control in our lives, which is an important factor in happiness. They also boost our self-esteem.

## A Boost to Self-esteem

Kindness makes us all happier but it can make some of us *very* happy. This was the outcome of some research published in the *Journal of Happiness Studies* that involved 119 Japanese women (71 in a kindness group and 48 in a control group, for comparison).

Unlike some kindness studies, where people are asked to go out and perform acts of kindness, the women in this study were simply asked to notice their own behaviour and record the number of kind acts they did each day and what they were. In effect, they were to *count* their kindnesses.

Simple though it was, 'counting kindnesses' had a large impact on the women's lives: they basically all became happier. But for 20 of the women (around 30 per cent of the 71 in the kindness group), the exercise had a significant effect: they became *much* happier.

I believe this was because it boosted their self-esteem. I've noted this when I've encouraged people to try this exercise. When they count their kindnesses, many people arrive at the conclusion that they are much kinder people than they thought they were, and they suddenly realize that they make more of a contribution to other people's lives than they previously imagined. For some, this is just the boost their self-esteem needs and they have a greater sense of value and purpose as a result.

One person explained to me that when he was younger he'd been told that he wasn't a nice person. The idea had somehow stuck. When he did this exercise, he was quite overcome by the realization that he made more of a difference than he thought.

'It was the small things that came in large numbers,' he commented, 'that made the biggest difference.'

## ACT OF KINDNESS

*Buy an extra parking ticket and
leave it on the parking meter for
the next person to find.*

When we think of acts of kindness, we may imagine we have to do something big, something significant and noticeable, perhaps something that even requires some planning, but for this man it was the realization that each day is filled with dozens of small kindnesses – holding a door open, listening, picking up a dropped pen, smiling at someone, nodding in agreement to make someone feel validated – that made the big difference. For him, these were the kindnesses that counted most.

## Giving Makes Young Children Happy

My youngest sister, Lynn, who is six years younger than me, inspired me when she was a child. I was often moved by her willingness to give me or one of my other sisters whatever she had – sweets, toys and even money.

The kindness of children is something that scientists have studied a lot. One piece of research, conducted at the University of British Columbia in Canada, investigated what happened when toddlers under the age of two gave away toys or sweets.

Two trained assistants observed the toddlers and used their facial expressions and other cues to evaluate how happy they seemed to be. A smile was listed as a positive while a frown was a negative, for example.

The toddlers were playing a game with a puppet, something often used in research to study children's moral behaviour under controlled conditions. During the game, they were occasionally given treats. The question was, would they be happier receiving the treats themselves or giving them to the puppet?

You guessed it! They were happier when they gave treats to the puppet than when they received them themselves. Not only that, but they were happier even when they gave up the chance of receiving a treat themselves so that the puppet could receive it.[5]

What does this tell us? Children like to receive. Of course they do. But they also like to give.

I remember as a child at Christmas time hearing my mum say she got more pleasure out of giving presents than receiving them. I couldn't get my head around that. I loved getting presents at Christmas. I could barely sleep the night before out of pure excitement.

But at the same time, one of my most significant childhood memories, one that filled me with real pleasure, was giving presents to my mum and dad. One year I gave Mum a Cadbury's Flake chocolate bar that I'd bought for her with my pocket money and I gave Dad half a dozen of his own dominoes wrapped in a piece of paper. I was probably only about four years old at the time.

As we've recalled that memory over the years, my mum has always impressed upon me that 'it's the thought that counts'. It's not so much *what* you give that matters, it's the *thought behind it* that's most important. And because you are giving something, that thought will always be one of kindness.

## Kindness Can Reduce Social Anxiety

Social anxiety is worry or fear of being in certain situations. It can erode our confidence and happiness. We worry that we might not be able to keep up a conversation, that we might get nervous, sweat, blush, be embarrassed, be humiliated in some way, be rejected. We become acutely concerned with what people might be thinking about us. We may even get nervous at the *thought* of having to be in some situations.

### ACT OF KINDNESS

*Pay for an extra pair of cinema tickets and ask the server to give them to someone they feel would appreciate them.*

John was a socially anxious friend of mine at school. He seemed happy enough when he was with close friends or people with whom he felt safe, but when there were more people around, especially the 'in crowd', he would become very quiet.

I remember he helped me once with my English homework and explained the meaning of some words that I didn't understand. He was intelligent. But his anxiety around people made him more and more withdrawn. He was teased – I remember one kid would call him 'Failure' instead of John – and he left school at the earliest opportunity. I often wonder what became of him.

Lots of people experience social anxiety and it can really dent their happiness, a) because a lot of happiness comes from interaction with people and b) because they spend a lot of time focusing on their fear of being in certain places. But recent scientific research indicates that kindness is a very powerful intervention for people with social anxiety.

In a four-week study at the University of British Columbia, 142 volunteers with high levels of social anxiety were randomized to either perform acts of kindness, participate in behavioural experiments or be in a control group. At the start of the study and every week throughout, they reported on their mood, anxiety levels and social activities.

Those in the kindness group experienced significant improvements in positive emotion throughout the study and even after the four weeks had elapsed. They not only felt happier, but their relationships improved, they became more confident and they tended to avoid some social situations much less. Kindness had made them happier *and* more socially comfortable.[6]

## An Antidote to Depression

Margaret McCathie suffered from depression. 'It was so bad,' she said, 'that I made a few suicide attempts.'

> *Once I was kept in a locked ward for a month. The staff were not very nice. There was little kindness. No compassion at all! I think mental health is generally misunderstood.*
>
> *I was given electroconvulsive therapy. It didn't work. I think it did more harm than good.*
>
> *One day I decided I couldn't take any more and threw myself off a waterfall into a fast-flowing river. Then my bum got stuck between two rocks and it stopped me from drowning!*

Recalling the incident, she literally burst out laughing. The laughter came from the fact that she is in a very different place today.

'What happened?' I asked. 'What helped you out of your depression?'

> *I'd watched the film* Patch Adams, *featuring the late Robin Williams in the role of Patch. Patch is 'the laughter doctor'. He treats depression with laughter. So I sent him*

*a fax to ask if I could go to his hospital in the States, The Gesundheit! Institute.[7]*

*Patch sent a fax back the same day. The same day! This was in 1999 and he explained that the institute wasn't built yet. The advice he gave me instead was to 'Go out and serve and see your depression lift.'*

*Within a month I had made a big improvement. Just knowing that he cared, his kindness – that made a huge difference to how I felt.*

*I followed his prescribed advice: I went out and served. My husband, Kenny, and I devoted ourselves to several hours of charitable work each month. We did 'Befriending', helping to support people with mental health problems by being there for them as friends. We did other charitable work, too. In my daily life, I simply took opportunities to help anyone in need.*

*It all helped. Love, the support of loved ones and kindness, to me and by me, played a big role in bringing me out of depression.*

Today, several years later, Margaret is a larger than life personality. She volunteers at a cancer charity once a week and runs workshops in prisons. She runs workshops for the public too, helping people to discover their 'wonderfulness'. In her experience, kindness equates to happiness.

The tendency with depression is to withdraw into ourselves. I understand it well, because I've suffered from it in my own life.

Focusing outwards, on helping others, is counterintuitive. The idea of giving to others when you're the one who needs help doesn't at first make sense. But when we do look outwards, towards the suffering or the needs of others, our natural tendency to care comes to life and the burden of depression can gradually dissipate.

At this point, the issue of whether helping others to make yourself happier is selfish or not becomes a non-issue. Try telling someone who is suffering from depression that they're being selfish by helping others. They certainly don't see it that way and nor do they care! Anything to find their way out of the dark! And kindness is one way.

## ACT OF KINDNESS

*Leave some money at the till of a coffee shop and ask the manager to use it to pay for everyone's coffees until it is used up.*

## A Legal High

Science wholeheartedly agrees with Margaret that the kindness of volunteering, of service, of helping others, makes us happier. Many people, in fact, get a high from doing good deeds for others. It's even been called 'helper's high', a term coined by Allan Luks in his 1979 book, *The Healing Power of Doing Good*.

Below are the results of a large US survey that Luks conducted of the health, happiness and volunteering habits of 3,296 people.[8]

| Percentage of the 3,296 people | How they felt when they helped someone |
|---|---|
| 95% | Felt good |
| 80% | Had positive feelings that stayed with them for hours (or days) afterwards |
| 57% | Had greater feelings of self-worth |
| 54% | Had an immediate warm feeling |
| 53% | Felt happier and more optimistic |
| 29% | Had more energy |
| 21% | Felt euphoric |

He basically showed that kindness makes us happier.

Part of the reason I've written this book is that although this is the experience of most people, surprisingly few make the connection between kindness and happiness and understand that they go hand in hand.

I've asked several people why they do kind things. One of the main answers I get (and it usually comes with a shrug) is 'Just because.' Kindness resonates at such a deep level with us that we don't even think about why we should show it. It's an inner feeling that says, 'Yep! This is how it's supposed to be.'

It's the 'rightness' of kindness and the connection that comes from it that feels so good. And this isn't a subjective feeling:

research suggests that kindness changes our brain chemistry. It boosts the levels of dopamine and serotonin, which are chemical messengers involved with positive emotions. It also produces oxytocin, the 'bonding hormone' (more on this in the next chapter). It even produces endorphins, the brain's natural versions of morphine and heroin. Kindness really does give us a totally legal high.

There are more benefits too, many of which you'll read about in this book. In summarizing much of the above study and some of his own personal observations, Allan Luks noted that helpers got fewer colds and less flu. They had fewer migraines. They slept better and overate less. Lupus sufferers who helped others had less pain. Asthma sufferers had some relief from their symptoms. Some patients who had had surgery even recovered more quickly.

The human body is wired for kindness. It's why kindness is beneficial for our health and makes us feel good. Later I'll show you how and why that is. For now, a little more on how kindness makes us happier.

## 'Moral Treatment'

As Margaret's experience showed us, kindness can help relieve depression. The most prescribed treatment for depression in our modern world is pharmaceutical, but it wasn't always that way. Kindness has been a treatment for depression and other psychiatric disorders for much longer.

'Moral treatment' began in the United Kingdom in 1796, when the York Retreat was founded by the Quaker William Tuke at Lamel Hill, York. Thirty depressed patients lived there as part of a small community. Receiving no medication or conventional therapeutic techniques at all, they were encouraged to build moral strength. Key to their recovery was service to others in the retreat.

The treatment was so successful that it spread to the USA and became widespread in the 1820s and 1830s. Psychiatrists were so convinced of the power of service that they believed that the methods led to 'organic changes in brain matter'.[9]

This knowledge has largely been forgotten and is ignored by mainstream medicine today. I believe that our society would be better off if we were to rekindle it. I'm not suggesting that we ignore pharmaceutical and other treatments, but if medical students and doctors could be taught that kindness can heal the heart and mind, and if people suffering from depression could understand that it can alleviate some of their symptoms, many patients, I believe, would benefit from a 'kindness prescription' as a primary course of action, or at least as a practice to be used in concert with other treatment.

Fortunately, some modern studies are in fact resurrecting this knowledge. It's even reaching government levels. In 2008 the 'Foresight Mental Capital and Wellbeing Project' was published by the UK Government Office for Science. It concluded that one of the '5 ways to mental wellbeing' was:

*Give... Do something nice for a friend, or a stranger. Thank*
*someone. Smile. Volunteer your time. Join a community group.*
*Look out, as well as in. Seeing yourself, and your happiness,*
*as linked to the wider community can be incredibly rewarding*
*and creates connections with the people around you.*[10]

In other words, *be kind.*

## A Tonic for Older People

Kindness is a great tonic for older people. A University of Texas study examined the mental health and volunteering habits of 3,617 adults over the age of 25. Those who volunteered, they discovered, had fewer symptoms of depression than those who didn't. But one of the key findings of the study was that the anti-depressant effect was even stronger in adults over 65 years of age.[11]

## ACT OF KINDNESS

*Tell someone in a shop or restaurant*
*that they're doing a great job.*

In a University of Wisconsin study, researchers examined data on the volunteering habits and health of 373 people between the ages of 65 and 74 that was collected in the 1995 National Survey of Midlife Development in the United States. They too found that volunteers reported less depression and more positive emotions than those who were not volunteers.[12]

Furthermore, a study of people over the age of 85 found a strong connection between altruism (that is, selfless concern for the wellbeing of others) and happiness. Studying the responses of 366 people to statements like 'I place the needs of others ahead of my own', it found that those who were most altruistic were happiest and had the fewest symptoms of depression.[13]

Being altruistic and placing the needs of others ahead of our own is not about neglecting our own needs, of course. It's not about saying, 'These people are more important than me.' Altruism is rooted in knowing that we are okay, not that we aren't as deserving as others. The former builds self-esteem, the latter erodes it. It's important to be aware of this.

As we get older, experience teaches us that altruism leads to happiness. We learn time and time again how good it feels, how right it feels, to help others, and so we learn to do more of it. For many, helping others is what gives their life meaning. It gives them a sense of purpose.

Indeed, kindness has been shown to give older people a greater will to live. A study compared volunteers over 65 years of age to retired people of the same age group who didn't volunteer. Those who volunteered were found to be much more satisfied with their lives. They had fewer symptoms of depression, anxiety and somatization (which is where psychological states are expressed in the body as physical symptoms), and a stronger will to live than those who didn't volunteer.[14]

This is important because some people who reach retirement don't feel useful any more. Often they lose the connections they enjoyed with their work colleagues and friends. This kind of research can encourage older people who feel this way to reach out to others as well as create some much-needed social contact again.

## Out of Your Comfort Zone

I've been writing and speaking about kindness for years. Sometimes I suggest to people that they push themselves out of their comfort zone in an effort to be kind. These efforts often bring big rewards. Sometimes the same thing happens to me.

For instance, a few years ago I learned that my P7 schoolteacher, Mr Hooks, who taught me when I was 11 years old, was still teaching in the same school. It was now attended by my niece, Ellie, and one day I went with my mum to collect her after school and Mum arranged for me to go and see him.

I remember feeling so nervous. I was like an 11-year-old again. Would Mr Hooks remember me? Of course he wouldn't. It had been more than 30 years since I'd been in his class.

But when the head introduced us and Mr Hooks got my name, he did remember me and how I'd done so well in maths.

I then plucked up the courage to say what I'd come to say. I thanked him for being such a good teacher and for instilling in me a love of maths and science, and I thanked him for allowing me to work at my own pace in maths. I'd been a bit of a geek back then – I used to take my maths textbook home at night and work through extra examples and problems. Now I told Mr Hooks I was grateful that he'd given me the freedom to do this.

I also relayed how well I'd done at university and how I'd worked as a scientist, and said that I was glad that I'd had him as a teacher. I told him he'd helped shape the learning choices I'd made and ultimately the direction I'd taken in life. I then gave him a signed copy of my latest book.

I wasn't sure at that point how he felt. A little taken aback, perhaps. I even got the sense that he was a bit embarrassed, not sure how to respond. He introduced me to the class as a former pupil and we then chatted a bit about his upcoming retirement.

A month or so later he e-mailed after spending a family holiday in Canada. One evening over dinner, he'd told his family about my visit. He wrote that he'd felt like the 'king of the castle' and they'd all been very impressed. And he added that he'd been quite touched to learn that he'd had such a positive influence on a student's life.

I'm sharing this personal example not because I want to impress you, but because I want to impress *upon* you that kindness sometimes really matters for the people we help.

I was out of my comfort zone when I went to meet Mr Hooks, but it was so worthwhile. As well as making him feel good, this act of kindness lifted my spirits for days afterwards. That wasn't why I did it. I hoped that it would help make Mr Hooks' day. But it made me feel good just the same.

So, what about your own life? How can you leave your own comfort zone and be kind?

## ACT OF KINDNESS

*When someone cuts you up on the road, smile and wave them on.*

## Physical Changes in the Brain

Some people like to meditate on kindness. Buddhists are fans of this. The loving-kindness meditation is a Buddhist exercise that helps us develop our sense of kindness and compassion. Buddhists have been practising it for centuries, but it has recently received attention in the West and has been studied because of its health-giving effects.

Some research suggests that it actually creates physical changes in the brain, both on the left-hand side of the prefrontal cortex (the bit above our eyes), which is often thought of as the seat of positivity and compassion, and in a region known as the *insula*, which is considered to be the empathy centre.

Stop and think for a moment: we're not simply talking of how kindness makes us feel good, we're talking about *physical changes in the brain* as a consequence of thinking about being kind and compassionate, feeling the warm, uplifting feelings of kindness and compassion and taking the appropriate action.

A story goes that scientists travelled to a Tibetan Buddhist monastery to study the brains of the monks there who practised the meditation. But when they connected their apparatus to the monks' brains, they couldn't get a proper reading. The dial seemed stuck. Assuming that their equipment had been  damaged during their travels, they eventually had to contact the university back in the States and have new parts shipped out to Tibet.

However, the new equipment behaved in the same way. It was only when one of the scientists tried it on himself that they discovered that the dial wasn't stuck at all. It had only appeared that way when they wired up the monks because the power output of the monks' brains was so high it had 'stuck' the dial on 'maximum'. In order to get a proper reading, the scientists had to recalibrate their equipment.

The high reading from the monks' brains was believed to be due to dense wiring in different parts of their brains as a result of their practice of compassion.[15]

It was also notable that the monks seemed to be very happy and laughed a lot.

## ACT OF KINDNESS

*Do a chore for someone that*
*you know they hate doing.*

In the West, the loving-kindness meditation has now been extensively tested for happiness- and joy-inducing qualities. One such study was led by psychologist Barbara Fredrickson of the University of North Carolina at Chapel Hill and involved 139 people who practised it daily for seven weeks.

The results were quite startling. There were increases in the participants' daily experiences of positive emotions, which included love, joy, gratitude, contentment, hope, pride, interest, amusement and awe. As a consequence, they felt more optimism, a greater sense of purpose and more mastery over their lives, they enjoyed improvements in the quality of their relationships and they experienced better health and a greater sense of life satisfaction.

Another benefit of the experiment was that positivity begat positivity. The increase in positive emotions felt after each week of meditation actually increased with practice. In the first week, the increase was 0.06 units for each hour of meditation, but after seven weeks' practice, one hour of meditation equated to 0.17 units' increase in positive emotions, an indication of physical brain changes.[16]

Meditating on kindness and compassion made it easier to practise kindness and compassion and, in turn, the participants derived more benefits from doing so. And the key was that some of these benefits occurred because the feelings brought about by kindness and compassion caused physical changes in the brain.

# Compassion Increases Happiness

*He who has mercy for the poor, happy is he.*

Proverbs 14:21

Compassion is like going into someone's suffering, sharing it with them and wishing them relief from it. It comes just before kindness.

I think of the evolution of empathy into compassion and then kindness as like a seed growing into a flower:

*Empathy* is 'I feel *with* you': I see your pain and share it with you. Empathy is a seed that grows into the stem of compassion.

*Compassion* feels bigger. It encompasses empathy, but adds the conscious wish that you be free of your suffering: 'I feel your pain, I'm with you, but I want you to be free of it.' It even adds a willingness to help.

The stem then grows into a full flower of *kindness*, which is the heartfelt approach that grows out of compassion.

In a compassion study led by researchers at York University in the UK, 719 people either took compassionate action for one week or were in a control group. Those in the group taking compassionate action were asked to act compassionately towards people they perceived to be suffering, for example to speak to a homeless person.

Over the next six months, those who had practised the compassion became happier and their self-esteem grew. The kindness of the compassionate action had produced happiness.[17]

This tallies well with HH the Dalai Lama's words, 'If you want others to be happy, practise compassion. If you want to be happy, practise compassion.'

Just as focusing on helping others helps alleviate depression, having compassion for the suffering of others takes us out of our own suffering. It stops us focusing on the problems that are causing us worry and stress. It aligns us with our deepest nature. It lets us glimpse a grander part of ourselves, that portion that genuinely wants to see our friends and loved ones happy, and that is happy itself.

## The Kindness of Gratitude

**Gratitude [*grat-i-tjud*]:** The quality of being thankful; readiness to show appreciation for and to return kindness. Counting blessings.

Elizabeth and I bought our first home last year after renting for nine years. It was a big step.

Being completely inexperienced, we didn't really know what we were taking on when we bought an old cottage. I honestly thought it just needed repainting and a new kitchen, but it turned out that it needed new electrics (a complete rewire, due to its age), a new boiler and a complete repiping (due to the age of the pipes), a few new walls, new beams and floorboards in one of the rooms, a full replastering before painting, restoration of the original shutters, restoration of the stairs, new windowsills, new doors, door facings, flooring, and many other bits and pieces. Oh, and a new kitchen, of course. At least I got one thing right.

My friend Kenny, a retired carpenter, gave me some tools, cut our kitchen worktop, and showed me how to cut and fit skirting boards. We had professionals who did the electrics, plumbing and plastering, but, with the help of family, we did the rest of it ourselves. I'd changed a couple of lightbulbs in my life and wired a plug (badly). Now I was building stud walls and doing just about everything you can imagine in a full-time renovation that took six months. My dad worked with me almost every day as we figured out how to do most of the jobs that needed doing, while my Uncle John, a retired painter and decorator, helped with painting and taught Elizabeth all she needed to know to decorate the interior. He also instilled in me the belief that anything could be fixed! My mum and sisters, meanwhile, pitched in everywhere they could.

Elizabeth's mum and dad gave us a roof over our heads during this period when our house was uninhabitable and provided us with meals. Elizabeth's mum also washed all our clothes, which were always caked in dust.

I am filled with intense gratitude for all of the things that my mum and dad, my Uncle John, Elizabeth's mum and dad and the professionals, most of whom were family friends or the family of friends, did to help us. Each time I think back to those months and the kindness of everyone involved, I feel a little burst of warmth and happiness as I experience the gratitude for all that they did. I also have an overwhelming wish to do something to help them – to reciprocate in some way.

That's what gratitude does. It makes us feel good inside and creates a desire to do something in return.

And I find that the more we focus on things we're grateful for, the more things we find to be grateful for. Gratitude is a practice that improves with practice. And it definitely makes us happier.

I'm not just saying that – it was also the conclusion of a 10-week study involving 192 people that was conducted by psychologists at the University of California at Davis and the University of Miami in 2003.

Once a week the participants had to write down either five things that they were grateful for (the gratitude group) or five hassles (the hassles group) or just five general things that had happened in the past week (the control group, for comparison). The study has been called a 'blessings vs burdens' study.

Some of the examples given by the gratitude group included 'being grateful to God for giving me determination', 'wonderful parents', 'the generosity of friends', 'for waking me up this morning' and even 'for the Rolling Stones'.

Some of the examples in the hassles group included, 'finances depleting quickly', 'stupid people driving', 'a messy kitchen that no one will clean' and 'doing a favour for a friend who didn't appreciate it'.

At the end of the 10 weeks, those in the gratitude group were much happier than those in the hassles group. Compared with the control group, gratitude made people happier and focusing on hassles made people unhappier.[18]

The scientists also did a two-week study as part of the same research. This time, 157 participants did a gratitude exercise every day for the two weeks. Again, the happiness and wellbeing of those in the gratitude group became much higher than those in the hassles group.

The study also included a few extra measures of overall wellbeing. One was how much positive emotion the participants felt. Those in the gratitude group enjoyed significantly more positive emotion in their daily lives than those in the hassles group. In general, participants in the gratitude group were more joyful, excited, energetic, enthusiastic, determined, strong, interested and attentive than those in the hassles group.

And according to the testimony of friends and family members of the participants, those who did the gratitude work became more thoughtful and kind.

So gratitude is a great practice for improving happiness all round.

## Light and Dark

'What about when times are hard?' many people ask. 'It's much harder to be grateful then.'

I completely agree. When times are hard, often the only thing we can do is just get through them.

Gratitude doesn't ignore difficult times, nor does it pretend they don't exist. A regular practice of gratitude merely trains the mind to scan the everyday landscape of our life and settle more on the light than the dark. That's all. And as it settles on the light, it makes us feel better.

### ACT OF KINDNESS

*Give someone a compliment.*

We can take some inspiration from a study of the relatives of people with Alzheimer's, led by psychologist Jo-Ann Tsang of Baylor University in Waco, Texas. Half wrote down what they felt grateful for each day in a 'gratitude journal' and half made a list of their daily hardships. At the end of the study, those who wrote in gratitude journals reported greater overall wellbeing and also less stress and depression.[19]

One of the things the study found was that some of those in the gratitude group began to celebrate small victories, like being called by name by the Alzheimer's sufferer, for instance. Without a practice of gratitude, such a small thing might not have felt as meaningful.

In the stresses and worries that saturate our minds when we are under pressure and feel overwhelmed, these small things almost always go unnoticed. But given some attention, they can actually sow the seeds of a little extra happiness.

## The Power of Kindness

So far, we've learned that being kind makes us happier, but of course it also makes the people we're kind to happier, too. It can literally transform lives.

We often never know the impact of an act of kindness or compassion on another person. Sometimes it can leave a lasting impression.

I was working in a bar once and Jack was one of the regulars. He was a kindly man in his mid to late seventies, I presumed, and he would come in every day at lunchtime and order a Bell's whisky. One day he told me this story:

> At one point during World War II, I got separated from my company. I was in a small town filled with bombed-out buildings. Some German soldiers were approaching and searching the buildings. I was terrified. If they found me, they would kill me.
>
> I tried my best to stay totally quiet. I was even scared to breathe in case anyone heard me.

*When the soldiers reached the building I was in, I was shaking with fear. I've never been so terrified in my life. I could hear someone really close. I grasped my gun, but I couldn't think straight.*

*Then he saw me. He was staring right at me with his gun raised. I didn't raise mine – I was too scared.*

*Then I lost control and wet myself, right there in front of him.*

*He looked at me for a moment, then he took me completely by surprise. He squinted his eyes a little, then gave me a compassionate smile and a gentle nod, and walked away, signalling to the other soldiers that the building was clear.*

*I've never forgotten that. It's the thing I remember most about the war.*

I've never forgotten that either. Overcoming the hatred of war and sparing the life of an enemy shows true compassion.

Sometimes when an opportunity for compassion or kindness presents itself, we forget why we're supposed to judge or hate; we even forget our own suffering as something inside us rises to the surface and places someone's immediate needs above all else.

I am reminded of Victor Frankl, the Austrian psychiatrist who survived a Nazi concentration camp. In his book *Man's Search for Meaning*, he wrote:

*We who lived in concentration camps can remember
the men who walked through huts comforting
others, giving away their last piece of bread.
They may have been few in number, but they
offer sufficient proof that everything can be taken
from a man but one thing: the last of the human
freedoms – to choose his own attitude in any given
set of circumstances, to choose one's own way.*

We should never underestimate the power of a kind act, however big or seemingly small.

## Everyday Heroes

Small acts of kindness pepper most of our days – both little things we do ourselves and little things that are done for us. We may hardly notice them. They may seem small, at least in our own mind, but they all count. They all make a difference, even if that difference isn't obvious to us.

We don't need to change someone's life to 'qualify' as a kind person. The little things we do matter a lot because they are the things we do most often.

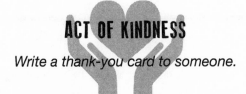

## ACT OF KINDNESS

*Write a thank-you card to someone.*

Everyone is an everyday hero in that respect. My mum is one. She has been kind every day I've been on this Earth, yet she probably wouldn't notice it. I once asked her when she'd last carried out an act of kindness and she couldn't think of one, yet she'd just made me a cup of tea and a sandwich! And that's the thing with everyday heroes: it's just their nature. Kindness is so natural to them that they don't even notice they're kind.

But the cups of tea, the looking after children, the lifts in the car, the hundreds of other things that family and friends do for each other every single day are all important. They're the glue that holds our relationships together. They're the threads in the fabric of our lives.

## CHAPTER SUMMARY

❤ Kindness can bring a smile to a person's face. But it also brings a smile to the face of the giver. It makes us all happier.

❤ Children feel happy when they're kind. Adults feel happy when they're kind. Older adults who volunteer to help others feel happier *and* have a greater sense of purpose and a greater will to live.

❤ Kindness can help relieve depression. It can boost self-esteem. It can reduce social anxiety.

❤ Kindness physically changes the brain. It produces serotonin, which is exactly what some antidepressants seek to boost.

It also alters the structure of the brain if we practise it consistently, essentially 'wiring in' a kind nature and the happiness that comes with it.

❤ Compassion and gratitude, both aspects of kindness in a broad sense, also improve happiness.

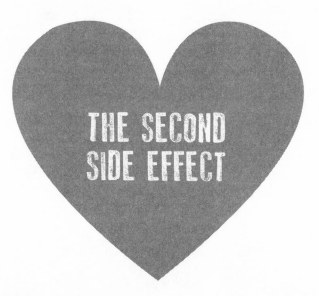

THE SECOND
SIDE EFFECT

# Kindness Is Good for the Heart

*Wherever you go, go with all your heart.*
CONFUCIUS

'A warm feeling in the chest!'

That's the most commonly reported physical sensation in relation to kindness. You've probably felt it yourself when you've been moved by witnessing or experiencing kindness.

Ever wondered what it is?

It's the effect of kindness on the heart.

The feelings brought about by kindness – warmth, elevation, inspiration, emotional connection – have a physical impact. Just as feeling embarrassed causes our face to flush and feeling excited speeds up our heart rate, so the feelings brought about by kindness have effects on the brain and body, especially the heart.

## The Love Hormone

In the first instance, kindness produces a hormone called oxytocin, and oxytocin is responsible for a whole range of positive effects on the heart and arteries.

Oxytocin is well known for its role in childbirth; it initiates uterine contractions and is the first choice medicine in many countries around the world for inducing labour. It was discovered by the British pharmacologist and physiologist Sir Henry Dale in 1906 and it was he who gave it its name, from the Greek words, ωκνξ, τοκοχξ, which mean 'swift birth'.[1]

It's also well known for its role in breastfeeding; it controls the 'letting down' of breast milk. Many women are given oxytocin in fact to help produce breast milk.

Oxytocin also plays a major role in helping mothers bond with their infants, parents bond with their children, siblings and friends bond with each other, adults bond with other adults, animals bond with animals, and humans bond with animals. It has a lot of nicknames and 'the bonding hormone' is one of them. Oxytocin is the glue that holds relationships and communities together.[2]

It's also responsible for feelings of trust; we tend to trust more when we have plenty of oxytocin. An increase in oxytocin will even make us like a person more. It turns down activity in the amygdala, a brain region that processes fear and anxiety. It's been shown to help reduce social anxiety. It even helps us understand each other's emotions.[3]

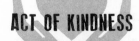

## ACT OF KINDNESS
*Adopt a dog from a dog shelter.*

It gets its popular name, the 'love hormone', because we turn on the oxytocin tap when we feel love, when we share warm emotional contact of any type and also when we have sex.

So important is oxytocin that it is on the World Health Organization's 'List of Essential Medicines', which are medicines considered of most importance in a basic health system.

It was always believed that oxytocin was produced in the brain and then secreted into the bloodstream. While this is true, recent research suggests that it is also produced in the heart.[4] Indeed, it plays a number of very important roles in the heart and throughout the entire cardiovascular system.

It's responsible for what's known as 'the Roseto Effect'.

## The Roseto Effect

Roseto is a town in Pennsylvania, USA, whose inhabitants participated in a scientific study lasting almost 50 years. During a census in the 1960s, it was found that not a single person in the town under the age of 45 had died of heart disease.

It was a startling find, given that the USA has the highest rate of heart disease of any country in the world. In Roseto, the death rate from heart disease even in over-65s was significantly lower than the rest of the country. It wasn't until 1970 that the first death from a heart attack was ever recorded there in a person under 55.

Scientists from around the world descended upon the town, sampling the water, studying the diet and even testing the atmospheric conditions. For years they couldn't find any logical reason why people in Roseto quite simply were not dying of heart disease.

But they eventually figured it out. After years of exhaustive research, including studying the residents themselves, they discovered that it was the close community bonds between the residents that protected them from heart disease.

One of the things that characterize a close community is people helping each other; which psychologists refer to as 'prosocial behaviour'. It's defined as 'any action intended to benefit another person, like sharing, cooperating, helping, giving' – i.e. kindness. And of course, oxytocin flows like a river under these conditions.

And when it's flowing, it is 'protective' of the heart – cardioprotective.

## Oxytocin: Cardioprotection

**Cardioprotective [car-dee-oh pro-tek-tive]**: Serving to protect the heart, especially from heart disease.

Lots of things are cardioprotective. Common sense tells us that exercise is cardioprotective. A person can also have a cardioprotective diet, like the Mediterranean diet, which is rich in fresh tomatoes, salads, fish and olive oil.

Oxytocin is a cardioprotective hormone, which also makes any feeling or action that produces it a cardioprotective feeling or a cardioprotective action. Therefore we can say that kindness is cardioprotective, love is cardioprotective and bonding with people and animals is cardioprotective, because kindness, love and bonding all produce oxytocin.

It's cardioprotection that saved the residents of Roseto from heart disease.

## ACT OF KINDNESS

*Use an online supermarket service
and send a box of food to a family
who you know could use it.*

How does it work?

Oxytocin causes cells along the walls of our arteries to relax. Then the arteries widen, or dilate, in what is known as vasodilation. This means three things: 1) that more blood can flow through the arteries; 2) that more blood flow can be delivered to the heart and other organs, and 3) that blood pressure is reduced. And reduced blood pressure ultimately means protection against heart attack and stroke.

I find it really quite cool how kindness can protect us from heart attack and stroke. The diagram below shows the process. Specifically, there are copious quantities of parking bays that are shaped for oxytocin lining the walls of our arteries. They are called 'oxytocin receptors', as they are *receptive* to oxytocin.

When oxytocin 'parks', it causes the cells in our arterial walls to make nitric oxide.[5] (Note that this is not nit*rous* oxide, which is the laughing gas that you get at the dentist, but nit*ric* oxide.) At the same time, the heart makes atrial natriuretic peptide (ANP) and delivers it into the bloodstream.

Nitric oxide and ANP are powerful vasodilators. So once they get into our arteries, our arteries dilate. This is the basis for the cardioprotective effect of kindness.[6]

So the chain of events – the internal domino effect, if you will – goes like this: kindness produces oxytocin, which produces nitric oxide and ANP, which dilate arteries and reduce blood pressure. This is how kindness is cardioprotective.

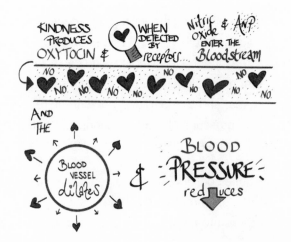

And we can substitute any feeling or method of producing oxytocin, like warm emotional contact, compassion, love, affection, sharing, sex, hugs, bonding with each other or animals, etc.

Now you can see why the residents of Roseto weren't getting heart disease.

## Kindness: Viagra for Your Arteries

Kindness is Viagra for your arteries. Literally! Viagra is really just a clever way to enhance the action of nitric oxide. It does it in the arteries that deliver blood to the penis, essentially increasing the flow of blood there.[7]

Nitric oxide is one of the most important substances in the human body. It's incredibly important for the heart and for the entire cardiovascular system. It's been called a 'miracle molecule' by Dr Louis Ignarro, who received the 1998 Nobel Prize for Medicine or Physiology for his work on it.[8]

Nitric oxide can prevent and even reverse cardiovascular disease. Our arteries produce it for the purpose of lowering blood pressure into the normal range and for improving blood flow to the heart, muscles and other organs.[9]

It also lowers LDL (bad) cholesterol levels and so helps to retain a healthy balance between the good stuff (HDL) and the bad stuff (LDL). In this way, it helps to prevent the build-up of plaque in our arteries that can lead to heart disease and stroke.

When nitric oxide is depleted, our arteries age much faster and blood flow is reduced to our muscles, organs and skin. In effect, when nitric oxide levels are depleted, we age faster on the inside.

So we can say that kindness really is like Viagra for our arteries. It perks them up and keeps them young and healthy.

# ACT OF KINDNESS

*Join a charity as a regular volunteer.*

## How Kindness Produces Oxytocin

Okay, so we know that the heart is pretty happy once we have plenty of oxytocin swimming about in our arteries. But how do we get it there in the first place?

Well, we are born with lots of it. It's vital for life. But the levels of it go up and down quite a bit and this depends on how we are *being*; i.e. kind or not.

Here are six common ways in which we produce oxytocin:

### 1) Through feeling elevated

'Elevation' is the word used by social psychologist Jonathan Haidt (pronounced 'Height') to describe the warm feeling we have when we witness an act of kindness or other demonstration of moral beauty. We turn on our oxytocin tap anytime this happens.

Typical responses to the question 'What makes you feel elevated, inspired?' include:

> 'I feel moved when I watch videos of happy dogs or of people helping others in difficulty. I always feel warm in my heart area and even get a lump in my throat sometimes.'

> 'When my husband is really busy, yet he still takes the time to make me breakfast in bed.'

> 'The video where the person buys food for the homeless guy and sits and talks to him for a while.'[10]

Even watching an inspiring video on YouTube, Facebook or any of the various media and social media channels available produces oxytocin. In fact, using videos like this is how scientists actually measure elevation in a controlled setting.

In a study led by Jonathan Haidt, for example, one group of breastfeeding women watched a morally uplifting film showing lots of kindness (to induce elevation in a controlled setting) and a separate group watched an equally enjoyable comedy video (as a control).

Observing the women afterwards, Haidt's team found those who had watched the morally uplifting film and experienced elevation were more likely to nurse their infants and more likely to hug them.[11] The urge to nurse an infant is very often triggered by the presence of oxytocin because, as we learned earlier, it controls the 'letting down' response of breast milk.

## 2) Comforting someone

Comforting also produces oxytocin in both the comforter and the comforted. One simple study found that a mother lovingly comforting her child produced oxytocin in the child.[12]

Even the anticipation of nursing an infant has been shown to produce substantial amounts of oxytocin in women.[13]

## 3) Warm emotional contact

Any kind of warm emotional contact, really, produces oxytocin. Think of how you feel when you witness or experience kindness, either as an observer, a giver or a receiver. You feel a warm connection, either with the people you are observing or as the person who is receiving or giving the kindness. It's this *feeling* – of elevation, inspiration, affection, emotional warmth, connection – that turns on the oxytocin tap. Even sharing food produces it.

## 4) Supporting a friend or loved one

You produce oxytocin any time you're there for a friend or loved one in need. Research by scientists from the University of North Carolina at Chapel Hill, for instance, showed that support from a partner was associated with higher blood oxytocin levels.[14]

The study involved 38 couples who were living together. They were asked to report on how much they supported each other, i.e. how much warm emotional contact they had. When the scientists measured everyone's blood oxytocin levels and cross-checked this with the reported levels of support given, those who had greatest amounts of oxytocin in their blood were the ones who had in fact reported the most amount of warm contact.

And unsurprisingly, the researchers also found that greater support equalled lower blood pressure in the 10 minutes after the warm contact.

Also, the more we give support, the more we benefit. The scientists pointed out that frequent positive interactions had cumulative long-term positive effects. Over time, they led to a sustained lowering of blood pressure.

### 5) Just thinking about it

But you don't need to actually be in a loving or kind situation to produce oxytocin, just as you don't need to be in a stressful situation to produce stress hormones.

Even just thinking fondly about someone you love, an experience of kindness or connection or a moment of warm contact produces oxytocin.[15] It's the feeling that does it. Women produce oxytocin just by thinking of their newborns.

### 6) Hugs

Hugs produce oxytocin too, but I'll leave this until later on, as I have a little more to say on the subject and I don't want to spoil it by telling you too early.

The point is that, as you can see, any time you're witnessing kindness, thinking about kindness, recalling kindness or performing an act of kindness, you're turning on your oxytocin tap. Essentially, oxytocin is a molecule of kindness.

## ACT OF KINDNESS

*Offer to look after a friend or family member's children for a few hours.*

## Kindness Softens Our Arteries

'As above, so below, as within, so without, as the universe, so the soul...' wrote the sage Hermes Trismegistus. The idea has a parallel in modern science in that our outward behaviour (kind or not) affects our inner health. Let me explain.

Hostility is thought of as an attitude of ill will and contempt towards people. A hardening, if you will. It is often expressed with anger. It is very far removed from kindness – an opposite of sorts, in terms of how we communicate with people.

Hostility is a significant risk factor for cardiovascular disease, just as kindness is cardioprotective. It might even be a more reliable route to cardiovascular disease than a bad diet.

A study at the University of Utah involved 150 married couples, who were asked to have a typical marital discussion while being videotaped. These videos were taken as indicative of the typical nature of the couples' relationships, so were indicative of a longer-term pattern.

When they watched the videotapes, the scientists categorized the couples according to how they behaved towards each other. At one end of the extreme were the couples who were most hostile towards each other and at the other end were those who were kindest and most loving.

Those who were most hostile were found to have high levels of 'coronary artery calcification', which is basically a hardening of the coronary arteries caused by a build-up of plaque. It's the difference between an artery with the internal consistency of a poached egg and one that feels like plasterboard. The couples who were the kindest and most loving had normal arteries.[16]

## ACT OF KINDNESS

*Buy some food for a homeless person.*

As we harden on the outside in our attitudes to people, so we harden on the inside in our arteries; as we soften on the outside in our attitudes to people, so we soften on the inside: 'As within, so without.'

The build-up of plaque that leads to hardening of the arteries is a consequence of two processes: oxidation and inflammation.

Kindness counters both. To understand how, you'll first need to understand a little about Harry Potter's spectacles.

## Harry Potter's Spectacles

Have you ever cut an apple in half and left it on the table? If so, you'll have noticed it quickly goes brown. This is oxidation.

Oxidation occurs in arteries too, and it can be a side effect of lifestyle and dietary stress. It doesn't happen as quickly in our arteries as it does in a sliced apple left on a table, so don't worry, but it happens nevertheless. It's caused by what are known as *free radicals*.

Here's a simple way to think of a free radical. Think of what Harry Potter's spectacles look like: two 'O's and a little bridge between them. His spectacles are actually the exact shape of *oxygen*, the stuff we breathe. Oxygen – $O_2$ – has two 'O' atoms and a *bond* (bridge) connecting them.

Now imagine Harry gets hit by one of Draco Malfoy's spells and it snaps the bridge of his spectacles. So now he has two single lenses that are no longer bonded to one another. When this happens to oxygen, not due to one of Draco's spells but to some kind of stress, the two 'O's are said to be *free radicals*.

Once bonded, they are now separate. Instead of being in a relationship, they are single. And they simply hate being single. They'll do anything to be back in a relationship.

Unfortunately, such is the strength of a free radical's desire to bond that it will happily covet its neighbour's wife, so to speak: it will pinch any nearby atom. This isn't so great for the body, especially if the atom pinched is part of the cells that line our arteries, or our immune system, or a skin cell, or a brain cell. Once the free radical has taken their atom, these cells can begin to fall apart.

The body has natural ways of dealing with free radicals, though. It uses anti-oxidants. An anti-oxidant is anti (against) oxidation. It is a willing partner for a free radical, thereby eliminating any further damage to cells.

We get anti-oxidants from many fruits and vegetables, salads, teas, cinnamon and dark chocolate. It's one of the reasons why doctors encourage us to eat those foods. We also have natural anti-oxidants in the body.

But when free radicals are produced more abundantly than the body is able to mop them up, that's when we get oxidation, or *oxidative stress*, as scientists prefer to call it.[17]

Oxidative stress plays a big role in cardiovascular disease. It's also linked with Alzheimer's disease, chronic fatigue, arthritis, Parkinson's disease and a number of other serious conditions. Combined with inflammation, it can cause hardening of the arteries.

Most people know what inflammation is. It's the redness and swelling that occurs after we get a cut or other injury. It's an important part of the initial immune response and helps to draw blood and nutrients to a wound site. But it also occurs on the inside of the body, in our arteries and joints and even around the cells of the immune system.

However, just as there are anti-oxidants to mop up free radicals, so there are ways to reduce excess inflammation, through natural anti-inflammatories and through the action of the vagus nerve. (More on the role of the vagus nerve in the next chapter.) But when inflammation overwhelms the body's ability to control it, we get what's called *persistent* or *chronic low-grade inflammation*. And, just like oxidative stress, it can be a consequence of diet, lifestyle, stress or hostility.

Added together, oxidative stress and inflammation can lead to plaques forming in arteries and that can lead to hardening of the arteries and then other diseases of the heart and cardiovascular system. This is where oxytocin comes in. It reduces oxidative stress and inflammation both in our arteries and throughout the immune system.

## ACT OF KINDNESS

*Phone someone up on their
birthday and sing 'Happy Birthday'
down the phone line to them.*

In a ground-breaking study, scientists at the Behavioural Medicine Research Centre and Department of Psychology at the University of Miami examined the effects of oxidative stress and inflammation on the cardiovascular system and the immune system. They took cells from blood vessels and from the immune system and put them under different forms of stress in the lab. This was meant to simulate the kind of stress that occurs inside the body. As expected, they then measured large increases in oxidative stress and inflammation.

Then they repeated the experiment, but this time they added oxytocin to the mix. Incredibly, the levels of oxidative stress and inflammation dropped quite substantially in both the blood vessel cells and the immune cells.

The conclusion was that oxytocin is both a natural antioxidant and a natural anti-inflammatory.[18]

So, since we produce oxytocin by being kind, we can confidently say that kindness is an antioxidant and an anti-inflammatory, as in:

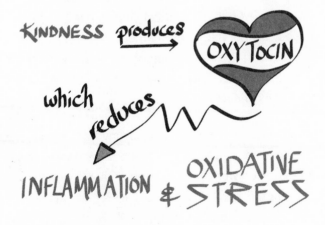

KINDNESS produces ➔ OXYTOCIN

which reduces

INFLAMMATION & OXIDATIVE STRESS

# The Power of Kindnnection

**Kindnnection [kaynd-nek-shuh n]**: A relationship in which one person or thing is connected to another, where the relationship is characterized by kindness.

Okay, that's a made-up word, but it means kind connections; that is, connections that are based on kindness, friendship or love.

Kindnnections are good for the heart. They provide emotional connection. They are essentially what the residents of Roseto enjoyed. Regardless of whether a resident of Roseto was single or in a relationship, it was kindnnections that protected them from heart disease.

A number of scientific studies have shown the same kind of thing. They also seem to have suggested that it is healthier to be married or in a relationship than to be single or living on your own. However, these kinds of studies need to be properly understood. It's not the being married or in a relationship that matters so much, it's the *quality* of the relationship that's the important thing. This is because a good-quality relationship turns on our oxytocin taps.

But we don't need to be romantically involved to enjoy good-quality relationships. We can have them with family or friends, neighbours or co-workers. We might interact with the person who delivers our post or with shop assistants. Many people's best relationships are with animals. All kinds of relationships count. As long as there's kindnnection, then the relationship is good for the heart.

This might come as welcome relief to single people who might have picked up the idea that only romantic relationships are good for the heart. It's fine to be single. 'Better to be single,' my friend Ann, who is a vet, joked, 'because you don't have to do someone's dirty washing.'

Joking aside, it's really about the connection – the *kind*nnection. And if you remember, kindness doesn't always require a physical act. It can simply be friendliness. It can be listening. It can be paying a compliment. It can be sympathy. It can even be laughing at someone's attempt to be funny, especially if it's not so funny (that's what my family and friends do for me). All these acts produce kindnnection.

Cardiologist Mimi Guarneri, author of *The Heart Speaks*, writes that cardiac patients benefit more from counselling and support groups (which involve kindnnection) than from the vegetarian meals they receive or the meditation or yoga that they are taught to practise.[19]

This is really quite amazing because most people have learned that having a good diet, taking exercise or reducing stress are the only ways to naturally benefit the heart. And it's also welcome news to the ears of people who feel guilty, perhaps, because they don't do the whole green living and yoga thing. Kindness and human (and animal) connection do a lot of good regardless of lifestyle, as the residents of Roseto would tell you.

Furthermore, in her book, Dr Guarneri suggests that some heart patients get a dog. This isn't just for the exercise, which of course is beneficial, but for the kindnnection.

## Being Kind to Animals

Forming kindnnections with animals is very good for the heart. Studies show that people who have a dog or cat in their family generally have lower blood pressure than people who don't have one. Blood pressure generally comes down when we stroke an animal.[20]

## ACT OF KINDNESS

*Offer your seat on the bus or train to an elderly person.*

In a study of 369 patients who had had a heart attack, the chance of a patient dying within a year was 400 per cent less if they had a dog than if they didn't have a dog.[21] Patients with a dog would have benefited from the exercise of walking and playing with the dog, but kindnnection would have played a major role, too. Interacting with and playing with the dog consistently throughout the day would have consistently elevated oxytocin levels and offered substantial cardioprotection.

Research has in fact shown that playing with dogs increases our oxytocin levels. In one study, conducted by scientists at Azuba University in Japan, 55 dog owners played with their dogs for half an hour. Oxytocin levels were taken at the start and again after the half-hour in both the human and the dog.

The scientists also videotaped the play sessions to examine the quality of the relationship each person had with their dog. They recorded how much time the dogs spent gazing at their owners and then split them into two groups. There were the 'long gazers', who made eye contact for an average of 2.5 minutes during the half-hour, and the 'short gazers', who only made eye contact for roughly 45 seconds. Long gazing was deemed to indicate a better quality of relationship between human and dog.

Oxytocin levels went up by 20 per cent in the long gazers compared with a control group of owners who didn't play with their dogs.[22]

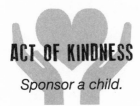

## ACT OF KINDNESS

*Sponsor a child.*

## An Antidote to Stress

*I was driving my car one day, heading towards the Forth Road Bridge, when I accidentally cut in front of another driver. He beeped his horn and hurled a number of expletives in my direction. He was really angry. He seemed to be having a bad day.*

*It was scary and upsetting, to be honest, but I gradually composed myself. When I eventually reached the bridge I was surprised to see that the same driver was now behind me again, right behind me as I drove into the tollbooth.*

*So I paid his toll charge for him.*

*About a half-mile further up the road, he drove alongside me. This time he had a large smile and greatly softened face and he mouthed the words, 'Thank you.'*

MAUREEN

There's no question that stress can cause heart disease. We've known this for decades. What we often miss is that kindness can diffuse stress, and the things that trigger it – anger, hostility and aggression, as well as worry, anxiety and fear.

Maureen's kindness neutralized the driver's anger and stress. She shared her story at a workshop I led. She told us that his anger left her feeling shaken, stressed and a little fearful. Yet right after paying his toll, she felt lighter and these feelings had gone. She felt a surge of positive emotion and a sense of connection with the driver instead.

Maureen's experience echoes a large body of scientific research that also shows that kindness counters stress. In a study led by Emily Ansell of Yale University School of Medicine, 77 volunteers received an automated phone call to their smartphones every evening for two weeks prompting them to fill out an online daily assessment. They were asked to record stressful events covering work, relationships, finances, health and other areas. They were also asked to record any kind acts they performed, such as holding open a door, helping someone with their homework, paying someone a compliment, etc.

Ansell found that those who reported more acts of kindness experienced less negative emotion and less stress. Even when some of them reported a number of stressful events, when there were also lots of little kindnesses on the same day, the stressful events had little or no impact on their emotions or sense of wellbeing. And on days when they didn't report as many kindnesses, they experienced more negative emotion in response to stressful events.[23]

Kindness neutralized the effects of stressful events.

In essence, as the level of kindness goes up in our lives, the level of negative emotion and stress comes down. And even when we experience stressful events, kindness can dampen the negative feelings.

In another study, people who were labelled as 'hostile' and who had chest pain were asked to wash one another's laundry. Incredibly, this simple act of kindness reduced their chest pain.[24]

It's funny how doing someone's washing can, in some ways, do the same as a heart drug.

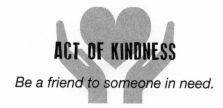

## ACT OF KINDNESS

*Be a friend to someone in need.*

## Thanks!

Gratitude is also cardioprotective, especially for people who have had a heart attack.

One of my friends had a heart attack a few years ago. I remember speaking to him about it. He took me by surprise when he said he felt grateful for it.

'Why?' I wondered.

He replied, 'Because it forced me to look at the way I led my life – my diet, my lack of exercise and especially my stress levels.'

Research has found that gratitude really does help people with heart conditions. In a University of Connecticut study, psychologists found that heart attack patients who saw benefits from their heart attack, which might include appreciating life more or seeing it as a gift, for example, were much less likely to have another heart attack over the next eight years than those who blamed their heart attack on others.

Those who blamed had a much higher risk of having another heart attack.[25] Seeing benefits in their experience was protective. Blaming was destructive.

In another study, scientists asked 3,000 patients with significant coronary artery blockages if they counted their blessings and had social support. It found that those who were the most grateful in their lives and had the most social support (opportunities to turn on their oxytocin taps) had the fewest blockages.[26]

## A Hug a Day Keeps the Cardiologist Away

Hugs are a natural expression of kindness, love, affection and gratitude. They can break down barriers between people. A hug can ease pain, both emotional and physical. Parents hug their children. Husbands hug their wives. Wives hug their husbands. Same-sex partners hug each other. Friends hug each other. Siblings hug each other. Some people who hardly know each other exchange hugs as greetings. People even offer 'Free Hugs' on the streets. Many people hug dogs, cats, horses and other animals. Some even hug trees.

Most of us enjoy hugs. They bring us closer together – not just physically but emotionally, too. They also produce oxytocin.

## ACT OF KINDNESS

*Make a donation to a charity.*

In one simple study, scientists at the University of North Carolina at Chapel Hill compared the number of hugs a group of 59 women received over a period of a month. Then they measured each woman's levels of oxytocin.

What was the result? The women who had the most hugs also had the most oxytocin. Simple as that! They also had the lowest blood pressure and heart rates.[27]

So we can truly say that a hug a day keeps the cardiologist away!

On 17 October 1995, twins Kyrie and Brielle Jackson were born 12 weeks premature in Worcester, Massachusetts, Boston, weighing in at around two pounds each. Over the next few days, Kyrie gained weight, but Brielle struggled. Sometimes she would cry and cry until she was gasping for breath and her face was turning blue.

On one really bad day for Brielle in the Neonatal ICU, 19-year-old nurse Gayle Kasparian was trying everything to settle her, but nothing was working. Brielle was in a really bad state.

But then Nurse Kasparian had an idea. With the permission of the parents, she took Kyrie out of her incubator and placed her into Brielle's incubator, something that was against the hospital's standard practice. Separate incubators were always used to reduce the risk of cross-infection.

Then a miracle happened. As doctors and nurses watched, little Kyrie moved her arm and placed it around Brielle, apparently hugging her tiny sister.

Almost immediately, Brielle began to get stronger. Her heart rate stabilized, her heart started to beat more strongly, her temperature returned to normal, her very low blood oxygen saturation levels rose rapidly and she started breathing much better, in synch with Kyrie, turning from blue into a healthy pink.

Over the next few days, both twins grew stronger.

The hospital later changed its policy.

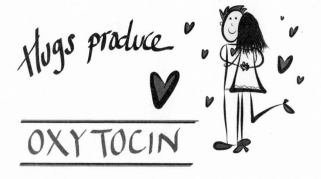

# CHAPTER SUMMARY

❤ Kindness uplifts us. Whether we witness it, receive it or show it, it produces a feeling of elevation.

❤ This feeling causes the release of oxytocin, which is a molecule of kindness, in our body. This, in turn, triggers the release of nitric oxide and ANP. The result is the dilation of our arteries and a reduction in blood pressure. Kindness is Viagra for our arteries.

❤ Nitric oxide also helps protect against the formation of the plaques that can lead to a heart attack or stroke.

❤ Oxytocin also counters two processes that lead to hardening of the arteries: oxidative stress (free radicals) and inflammation.

❤ So kindness protects the heart – it is cardioprotective.

❤ Being kind to animals is also good for the heart. It helps reduce blood pressure and having a dog significantly reduces the chances of a heart attack (by 400 per cent).

❤ Kindness is also an antidote to stress, so it can offset the risk that stress poses to our cardiovascular health.

❤ Hugs are good for the heart. A hug a day keeps the cardiologist away.

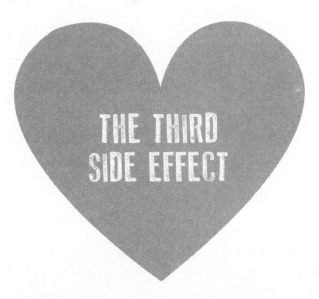

THE THIRD
SIDE EFFECT

# Kindness Slows Ageing

*You don't stop laughing because you grow old. You grow old because you stop laughing.*

MICHAEL PRITCHARD

What is ageing? In a nutshell, it is the process of getting older. It is seen in the all-too-obvious wrinkles on our faces, the degeneration of our muscles, the wear and tear in our joints, and our increasing susceptibility to illness, injury and disease. So, the best way to examine the slowing of ageing and the link with kindness is to look at these processes and see what being kind does to them.

Before we do that, you need to know that we have two ages: our *chronological age* and our *biological age*. Our chronological age is the number of years since our birth. It's the age we celebrate on our birthday. Our biological age, on the other hand, is the apparent age of our body, and it depends on a lot of things, including our diet, how much exercise we get, our stress levels, our attitude and whether we're kind or not. Our biological age can be younger or older than our chronological age.

## All in Your Genes?

'My great grandmother lived until she was 97, my grandfather to 93,' Rob declared proudly. 'My father is a still young 86. We have good genes in our family.'

'Mine aren't quite so lucky,' said Jane. 'My grandparents died from heart conditions in their seventies.'

Everybody knows that lifestyle affects health, but when we think of how fast our bodies age, most of us assume it's really all in our genes.[1]

Not wishing to take anything away from my friend with the apparently good genes, I agreed that it was likely he'd have around the same lifespan as his family members. However, I explained that it wasn't *all* down to 'good' genes.

Genetics only contributes around 20–30 per cent to longevity. So why do many members of a family line have similar lifespans? Well, the 20–30 per cent from their genes counts, of course. But as well as passing on genes, parents also pass on dietary habits, activity levels, attitudes, emotional style (how we respond to life's everyday stressors), behaviour and ways of connecting with people. And these habits make up a bigger fraction of the health equation than genes. They are what most determine our biological age and therefore how quickly or slowly our body ages.

Think about it. We learn a lot from our parents and grandparents. We learn which foods to eat by what they prepare for us. Healthy parents tend to produce healthy children who are more likely to grow into healthy adults. People with a sweet tooth usually have one or both parents with a sweet tooth. Parents who exercise are more likely to encourage their children to exercise than parents who don't. We also often learn to have the same level of self-esteem as our primary parent and this affects our emotional style and how we interact with others and form relationships.

Of course, we live in a diverse world and there are many exceptions. I am merely making some generalizations so that we can appreciate that it's not all about our genes.

Recognizing this makes it easier to accept that kindness can have an impact on ageing. Otherwise, if we surrender to our genes, it's all too easy to say, 'What's the point?' and do nothing about improving our health.

My friend whose family's lifespans seemed somewhat shorter than those of my other friend did proudly declare that her family had, on the whole, 'shocking' diets.

'And they don't exercise at all, except for walking around the shops,' she exclaimed in a somewhat relieved manner.

Did my other friend's family have a healthier lifestyle?

'Yes,' he said simply.

What this tells us is that our lifestyle, our attitudes to life and to other people, and how we treat others – with kindness or contempt, for instance – contribute quite a bit to the lifespan equation. There's a lot up for grabs in the longevity stakes, and the great thing is that our choices do matter.

## ACT OF KINDNESS

*Take out an advert in a newspaper*
*wishing everyone a nice day.*

## The Seven Big Agers

In this chapter, I'll discuss seven different processes of ageing and how kindness can slow them down.

The processes are: 1) muscle degeneration, 2) reduced vagal tone, 3) inflammation, 4) oxidative stress, 5) depleted nitric oxide, 6) shortening telomeres and 7) immunosenescence.

So, let's start with muscle degeneration.

### 1) Muscle degeneration

Most people point to the weakening and loss of muscle as being typical of ageing. 'It's just wear and tear. It happens when you get older.'

While this is true, few of us realize that how fast this process occurs has a lot to do with the exercise we take, the rest we get and the food we eat, plus our stress levels and our attitudes towards ageing and towards other people and animals.

Muscles do degenerate as we age, but they also *regenerate*. Muscle cells replenish themselves naturally and it is when the rate of degeneration is faster than the rate of regeneration that we have apparent ageing. That's why people who exercise stay fitter and stronger than people who don't, because exercise encourages muscle regeneration.

My friend Skip told me that he'd met a 98-year-old man in Bali who'd challenged him to a race to climb a tree. Skip is very physically fit – an ex-British champion gymnast in fact – yet the 98-year-old beat him.

I had a similar experience, in a way, when I spent six months of last year renovating our new home. It was almost a full-time job. First of all my dad and I had to remove the floorboards in one room, then get rid of all the large rocks underneath (typical in a very old cottage), so that a new floor could be laid.

Lifting the floorboards and removing the joists wasn't so hard. We did that in an hour or so. It was lifting the heavy rocks that was the hard bit. When I woke up the following morning, I could barely get out of bed. Muscles that I didn't even know existed were hurting. Walking to the shower and then downstairs for breakfast was very painful. I had to move with slow, deliberate steps.

Worried, I phoned my dad to see how he was. He was 73 years old, after all.

'Fine, son!' he replied, in an astonishingly (to me) upbeat voice. He was strolling around the kitchen making his breakfast. He wasn't in any pain at all.

How could that be? I'm in my mid-forties and absolutely no stranger to exercise. I used to be an amateur athlete and I still keep myself fit. How could Dad be completely fine when I felt … wrecked. I think that was the word I used that morning.

Quite simply, my dad spent 50 years in the building trade. Since he retired, he's been walking at least 50km (30 miles) every week. He's kept himself fit and that has ensured he's replenished lots of his muscle cells.

So, exercise is one way that our muscles regenerate. Can kindness help them regenerate too?

## ACT OF KINDNESS

*Offer to do some shopping
for someone who's not able
to do it for themselves.*

### How to get younger muscles

To replenish our muscle cells we need stem cells to grow into new muscle cells. You can think of a stem cell like a stem of a flower but lacking a head. It's basically just a stem. From this, it can grow any head, depending on its environment. In muscles, stem cells become muscle cells; in the brain, they become brain cells; in the heart, heart cells; and so on, all potentially from the same stem.

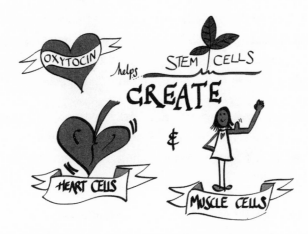

Scientists at the University of California at Berkeley were studying the regeneration of muscles when they made a very important discovery: stem cells don't convert to muscle cells very well at all when there's not much oxytocin.[2] If there's not enough of it flowing around, our muscles simply can't regenerate, so they weaken and age more quickly.

To regenerate our muscles, we need to have our oxytocin taps on.

And we're not just talking about the muscles that allow us to walk and lift objects – skeletal muscles – but the muscles in our heart too, according to some exciting new discoveries in science.[3] Oxytocin helps heart muscle cells grow from stem cells too, and when there's not much oxytocin around, *that* doesn't happen so well either.

So next time you have a hug or a loving gaze, think of how oxytocin is actually helping turn old muscles into young muscles – in your arms and legs, and also in your heart. Love and kindness, in effect, really can mend a broken heart. It's a pleasant thought.

When I explained this once, I had the following response: 'Surely it's really just that being kind is an antidote to stress, so kindness is just neutralizing the damaging effects of stress on our muscles?'

It's a fair point. Stress speeds up ageing and kindness counters stress, so kindness does slow ageing in that way. But the key here is that over and above countering the effects of stress, kindness acts *directly* on muscle regeneration at the cellular level.

## 2) *Reduced vagal tone*

The vagus nerve plays a very important role in slowing ageing. The word 'vagus' comes from the Latin for 'wandering', because this nerve literally wanders all over the body. 'It gets around' is how I described it to one woman. She raised her eyebrows. She's a relationship counsellor, so I can appreciate how she looked at it. But in 'getting around' the vagus nerve impacts a lot of systems in the body.

And just as we have muscle tone, which reflects the health and fitness of our muscles, so we also have vagal tone, which reflects the health and fitness of the vagus nerve. Vagal tone is typically high in children, but gradually reduces as we get older.

Why is this reduction in vagal tone important in ageing? Well, good vagal tone maintains the 'rest, digest and regenerate' mode in the body. It helps the body get the rest it needs, digest food so that it can be nourished and energized, and regenerate itself as wear and tear occurs. It also ensures that the vagus nerve can play its role in helping our organs work in harmony with one another.

We can therefore think of vagal tone as being protective against ageing. If it is low, we lose some of that protection.

## ACT OF KINDNESS

*Give your loved one breakfast in bed.*

You can see the vagus nerve at work for yourself if you take your pulse. Notice that your heart rate speeds up a little as you breathe in and then slows a little as you breathe out. The slowing as you breathe out is the vagus nerve sending your body into its rest, digest and regenerate mode. The difference in your heart rate between the in-breath and out-breath is a measure of vagal tone. The bigger the difference, generally speaking, the higher your vagal tone.

So, how do we increase vagal tone and therefore give our body more protection against ageing? Well, just as we can go to the gym and improve our muscle tone, so we can also exercise our vagus nerve and improve our vagal tone.

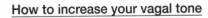

## How to increase your vagal tone

Vagal tone goes hand in hand with compassion and kindness. High vagal tone is associated with a broad range of compassionate and kind behaviour.

The link was first identified by Stephen Porges, of the University of Chicago, who saw a link between the vagus nerve and our social relations in what became widely known as Polyvagal Theory.[4]

In one example of how vagal tone is associated with compassion and kindness, a group of children watched videotapes of other children who had been injured in accidents and were now in hospital. All of the group had their vagal tone measured.

Afterwards, the children were given a chance to take homework to the injured children in hospital. Those who had the highest vagal tones were the ones who were most likely to volunteer to do so.[5]

In another study, conducted at the University of California at Berkeley, Jenny Stellar invited volunteers to watch a video of someone describing a sad event (a death in the family), or look at photos of people suffering (e.g. starving children) or watch videos of children with cancer. They were compared to a control group who watched a bland video (e.g. someone building a fence). Those who reported feeling most compassion were the ones with the highest vagal tone.[6]

The question is, given that high vagal tone is related to higher compassion and a greater tendency to be kind, and a low vagal tone is related to reduced compassion and less kind behaviour, can the *practice* of compassion and kindness actually increase vagal tone?

Indeed it can. Practising kindness and compassion is how we take the vagus nerve to the gym.

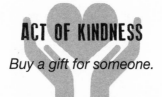

## ACT OF KINDNESS

*Buy a gift for someone.*

We briefly met the loving-kindness meditation in the first chapter. It's often called *mettā*, which is the Pali (the sacred language of Buddhism) term for 'loving-kindness'. It's defined as 'the wish that others find genuine happiness and wellbeing' and is rooted in an attitude of compassion and kindness. Scientists use it to study the effects of compassion and kindness under a controlled setting because everyone does the same meditation.

The meditator repeats a series of wishes such as: 'May [a loved one] be filled with loving-kindness, be well, peaceful and at ease, happy and free of suffering.' They focus these wishes on themselves, loved ones, random people, people who cause them some stress and all sentient beings (all life), in a gradually widening circle of compassion. With practice, this builds strong feelings of compassion and a motivation to be kind.

In a study conducted by psychologist Barbara Fredrickson and her team at the University of North Carolina at Chapel Hill, 65 men and women attended weekly loving-kindness meditation classes for six weeks and were encouraged to practise the meditation every day. They were compared to a control group who didn't do the meditation. Everyone's vagal tone was measured at the beginning of the study and again at the end.

After the six weeks, vagal tone had increased significantly in the loving-kindness meditators. It did not change at all in the control group. Practising compassion and kindness had directly increased vagal tone.[7]

## ACT OF KINDNESS

*Buy lunch or dinner for someone who is short of money.*

I have a lot of personal experience with this meditation. I practise and teach it often. I've learned that it builds *consistent* feelings of affection, compassion, goodwill and kind thinking. In effect, when we use it, our thoughts towards people gradually become softer not just during the meditation but in our general day-to-day life. I believe that this is what causes the gains in vagal tone.

Thus, the loving-kindness meditation isn't the only way in which we can increase vagal tone. Any way that we can develop our capacity for compassion and express it in kindness will increase vagal tone.

This again raises the issue about developing compassion in order to benefit ourselves. Are we being selfish? A Buddhist practitioner pointed out to me that compassion is to be developed for the benefit of all life. I couldn't agree more. That should be the primary purpose of developing compassion. But we're also talking about health. Once we know the link between vagal tone and compassion, we can't just pretend we don't know it, or not be compassionate lest we feel judged for being selfish. The cat is out the bag, so to speak.

To my mind, if we know that cultivating compassion that will ultimately benefit others also happens to be a way to improve our own health, that simply gives us a double reason to practise it.

## 3) Inflammation

As we mentioned earlier, inflammation is the body's reaction to a cut or other injury. It's a vital response of the immune system that helps draw blood, oxygen and nutrients to a wound site to help it to heal.

The problem with inflammation is that when there's more of it happening than the body can control, we get persistent (chronic) low-grade inflammation, where inflammation basically just keeps building up.

A friend trying to make sense of it once said, 'It's a bit like my children making mess in the house faster than my ability to clean up after them, so my house just gets messier and messier.'

Pretty much!

Her house getting messier is a good analogy, as it's the consequences of this kind of inflammation that we need to be careful of. You can think of it as being like a sink with a leaky tap dripping into it. The sink will eventually fill up and spill water onto the floor and the water will cause collateral damage to the floor and surrounding kitchen units.

In the same way, a persistent low-grade inflammation can build up and cause collateral damage to the heart, arteries, brain, skin and in fact all of the internal organs. It has been linked with almost all the serious diseases we know about, including cancer, heart disease, diabetes, arthritis, multiple sclerosis, frailty and Alzheimer's. In this way, it plays a major role in ageing. So much so that it has been called *inflammaging* by Claudio Franceschi, a professor in the Department of Experimental Pathology of the University of Bologna, Italy, who is an expert on the role of inflammation in ageing. It's even been suggested that if it weren't for inflammation, the human body would have the genetic potential to live to 150.[8]

Reducing inflammation is now one of the major approaches researchers are taking as they seek to find a drug to slow ageing.

**How to reduce inflammation**

The body does have its own process for controlling inflammation, though, just as my friend does the best she can to keep her house tidy.

It's the vagus nerve again, in what's known as the *inflammatory reflex*.[9] First discovered in 2002 by Kevin J. Tracey, a neurosurgeon and professor of neurosurgery at Hofstra Northshore School of Medicine in New York and president of the Feinstein Institute for Medical Research, it describes how the vagus nerve is the 'primary brake' on inflammation.

Think of your car, which has two brakes. There's the main brake, which you operate with your foot (the primary brake), and then there's the handbrake (the secondary brake), which you only ever use when you park your car or need to keep it from rolling down a gentle slope.

A high vagal tone basically equates to an efficient inflammatory reflex and therefore a good ability to keep the chronic low-grade inflammation and its collateral damage to a minimum.[10]

The loving-kindness meditation isn't only a good way to increase vagal tone; since the link between vagal tone and inflammation was discovered, scientists have extended the research to measure the effects of compassion and kindness directly on inflammation.

One study compared inflammation in 33 people who practised the loving-kindness meditation for six weeks with inflammation in 28 people in a control group who didn't do the meditation. After the six weeks, those who did the meditation had much lower inflammation levels than those who didn't. And those who did the most meditation practice had the lowest inflammation levels of all.[11]

# ACT OF KINDNESS

*If someone is giving out leaflets on the street, take one, smile and thank them for offering it to you. Make a point of reading it.*

## 4) Oxidative stress

Remember the story about Harry Potter's specs and free radicals?

Similar to the spill over of inflammation, we get oxidation (oxidative stress) when there are more free radicals than there is capacity to get rid of them. In arteries, this leads to plaques forming. In the brain, it leads to memory loss and difficulty concentrating. In the skin, it leads to wrinkles and the other visible signs of ageing.

This is why a number of facial products contain anti-oxidants – because they mop up free radicals. The face creams deliver the anti-oxidants right to the place where they're needed and they mop-up the free radicals there.

But to slow the formation of wrinkles and even remove some of the ones we already have, we only need to produce *natural* anti-oxidants.

This is where oxytocin comes in again.

## Smoothing out those wrinkles

Think for a moment of how skin ages under stress or emotional conflict. During these times there's a lack of oxytocin.

There's a connection here. It turns out that oxytocin plays an absolutely vital role in keeping our skin young and healthy. If there's not enough of it getting to the skin, the skin ages faster.

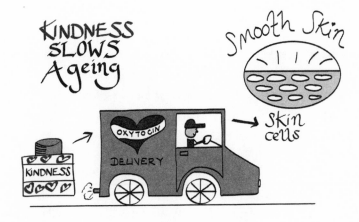

This was shown in research published in the journal *Experimental Dermatology*. Scientists were studying two types of skin cells: *keratinocytes*, which are the cells that makes up 90 per cent of the outer layer of skin, and *fibroblasts*, which are cells that make collagen. They basically found that as oxytocin goes up, free radicals come down in the keratinocytes and fibroblasts. The less oxytocin we have, on the other hand, the more free radicals we get.[12]

Oxytocin is *required* to keep our skin cells healthy and young. So when we're not keeping our oxytocin levels up through how we think about people and how we treat them, there's a risk that our skin could age faster.

'There's no way that just being kind is going to smooth wrinkles!' exclaimed a lady at one of my workshops. 'The mind might affect a lot of things, but it doesn't affect the skin! I'm a kind person, but I've still got wrinkles. That's just normal ageing!'

I can understand why she might think that. It does sound a bit 'out there'. We don't normally imagine that being kind can affect our skin. And wrinkles forming in our skin is a natural process of ageing, but, as I pointed out, how *fast* they form depends on our stress levels, our diet and also on how we are *being* (kind vs contemptuous, for example).

'Think of it the other way around,' I suggested. 'Notice how embarrassment turns your face red. A thought and the accompanying feeling alters blood flow to your skin. What about the way worry can turn your hair white? Or stress can age you? What about the way persistent anger can be etched on a person's face? These are all feelings and they all have a visible effect.'

Worry, stress and persistent anger age us because of the free radicals they produce and the oxidative stress they cause. Basically, kindness produces oxytocin and that 'molecule of kindness' mops up the free radicals in our skin. In this way, kindness slows the ageing of our skin.

# ACT OF KINDNESS

*If you are ever given too much change, take it back to the shop.*

On a separate note, our society has become a bit obsessed with ironing out wrinkles. The number of cosmetic surgery procedures has skyrocketed over the past few years. But here's the thing! Being kind in order to iron our wrinkles might not work. You see, oxytocin is only produced when kindness is genuine. If it's half-hearted in order to get a quick beneficial side effect, then that side effect won't happen.

So, don't make ironing out wrinkles your reason for being kind. Let kindness be the goal and just see what happens. Saturate your mind with positive ideas about people. Cultivate feelings of affection. Allow yourself to be uplifted by acts of moral beauty. You might be surprised at just how much this does for your skin.

### 5) Depleted nitric oxide

Nitric oxide is important in maintaining healthy blood pressure. It's also vital for maintaining healthy circulation, so that blood and nutrients can reach our muscles, skin, heart, lungs and brain. It helps to oxygenate our muscles, giving us more energy and endurance. It also helps to regenerate blood vessels, fight infection and keep our metabolism healthy. It aids the absorption of nutrients in the GI tract. It helps keep our memory sharp and our mind focused. It's no wonder Dr Louis Ignarro calls it the 'miracle molecule'.[13]

But nitric oxide levels tend to fall as we age, making this one of the key processes of ageing. It's partly why blood pressure tends to increase as we age. It's also why male sexual function can decline and why Viagra is so popular, as it boosts nitric oxide levels by stimulating the manufacture of nitric oxide in the penis. Depleted nitric oxide is also part of the reason why our muscles don't recover as fast after exercise, because they don't get enough flow of blood and oxygen. It's also partly why we become forgetful and have difficulty concentrating as we get older.

Not only this, but depleted nitric oxide is associated with many diseases of ageing.[14] Since nitric oxide plays such a critical role in maintaining blood pressure and circulation and combatting plaque formation, when levels are depleted, our risk of heart attack and stroke increases.

Lower levels also increase the risk of neurodegenerative diseases, including Alzheimer's. Research shows that amyloid plaques, the plaques believed to underpin Alzheimer's disease, are more likely to form in the absence of enough nitric oxide.[15] Keeping our levels up might be one of our best protections from dementia.

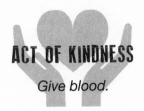

## ACT OF KINDNESS
*Give blood.*

Some scientists believe that keeping up our levels of nitric oxide is about the most important thing we can do to maintain our general health and slow ageing.

## Pump it up

Nitric oxide is a gas. There aren't actually bubbles of it floating around in our arteries, but it's a nice analogy because we can think of pumping up our levels.

Exercise is good for pumping up our nitric oxide levels. There are loads of foods that boost our levels too, including beans, coriander, watermelon, walnuts, pistachios, dark chocolate (for the cacao), pomegranates, spinach, kale, brown rice, beetroot, garlic and salmon.

I thought it would be useful to mention these here, but of course you'll be remembering the sequence from the last chapter:

*Kindness produces oxytocin, which produces nitric oxide.*

In short, kindness produces nitric oxide, which is, therefore, also a molecule of kindness.

In a simple study, just 20 minutes of the loving-kindness meditation was enough to significantly elevate levels of nitric oxide in a group of people who practised it.[16]

We know that the meditation helps us to feel compassion and dwell on kind sentiments, and it's these *feelings* that produce the nitric oxide. That's the key.

Just entertaining kind *thoughts* about people helps, or smiling at people, listening to them tell their stories, seeing the best in them and avoiding the temptation to focus on faults. All these things will boost our nitric oxide levels.

And nitric oxide doesn't just slow ageing. Some studies even suggest that increasing levels of nitric oxide might actually prolong lifespan, most likely due to the fact that it keeps our arteries healthy, blood pressure down and circulation at healthy levels.[17]

Nitric oxide really might be the 'miracle molecule', and we tap into that miracle through kindness, love, affection, compassion and elevation.

## 6) Shortening telomeres

Biological researcher Elizabeth Blackburn first discovered telomeres in 1976 and was awarded the Nobel Prize in 2009 for the discovery. Such is their importance that in 2007, Blackburn made *Time* magazine's list of the 100 most influential people in the world.

Telomeres are end caps on DNA that stop it unravelling when cells divide. A good analogy is to think of them as being like the plastic end caps on our shoelaces. Once they wear away, we can no longer use the shoelace because we can't thread it through the hole. In a similar way, once the telomeres wear away, DNA unravels and the cell dies. This is why telomeres are so important in ageing. Telomere length is, in fact, one of the most accurate ways of measuring biological age. And slowing the wear and tear on them is a powerful way to slow ageing at the genetic level.

## Building up our telomeres

So, how do the telomeres wear down? Well, it's down to the usual culprits really: stress, diet, lifestyle, attitude and behaviour.

Several studies show that people under stress tend to have shorter telomeres. Stress can also be a consequence of attitude. A positive attitude in the face of everyday stressors – the kind of day-to-day inconveniences that we all have – helps us get by with less stress. And acts of kindness, even on stressful days, as we learned earlier, helps keep stress levels low.

Kindness spares us a lot of stress and therefore, by extension, also impacts the length of our telomeres.

Family environments can be an early source of stress for many. The AIM (Adults in the Making) programme, which sets out to replace stress with emotional support and kindness, is based on the idea that positive, supportive family relationships are healthy.

In a study at the University of Georgia's Center for Family Research, 216 African-American high school youths had their telomeres measured at the start of an AIM programme when they were 17 years old and again five years later.

There were six weekly training sessions in which the youths learned how to make plans for their future and also how to identify people in their community who could offer them practical support, emotional support and guidance in dealing with problems, which included racial discrimination.

Their parents were also given weekly training sessions that helped them to develop a range of skills, including how to support their children emotionally and practically. Each week also had a joint parent–child session, which was about helping parent and youth to understand each other better and to bond. Ultimately, the programme brought more kindness, emotional support and emotional bonding into the lives of the youths.

When their telomeres were measured five years after the sessions began, they had shortened in the control group, which hadn't received the AIM training, yet they hadn't changed at all in the group that had received the AIM training.[18]

Kindness and higher levels of warmth and emotional support, along with practical guidance and problem-solving skills, had protected the youths against the loss of telomere length and had in effect slowed their rate of ageing.

The importance of kindness and emotional support in the lives of young people (and people of all ages) cannot be overstated. Clearly, it impacts them at the genetic level.

## ACT OF KINDNESS

*Write a letter of gratitude to someone who has influenced your life, deliver it by hand and read it out to them.*

In a different kind of telomere study, conducted by Elizabeth Hoge at Massachusetts General Hospital, 15 experienced loving-kindness meditators and 22 people of the same age who weren't meditators had their telomere lengths measured.

The experienced meditators had been practising the meditation daily for at least four years, clocking up an average of 512 hours of feeling sentiments of love, affection, compassion and kindness. Hoge found that they had much longer telomeres than the non-meditators, and that the effect was especially pronounced in female loving-kindness meditators.[19]

In effect, the warm feelings of love, affection, compassion and kindness that the meditation created protected their telomeres against everyday wear and tear.

In both these telomere studies, emotional warmth, emotional support, love, kindness and compassion – all aspects of kindness – had slowed ageing at the genetic level.

### 7) Immunosenescence

**Immunosenescence [I myune o sen eh sense]:** The gradual weakening of the immune system that occurs with age.

The immune system is the network of cells, tissues and organs that helps protect our body from infection and disease. It gradually weakens with age, making us more prone to illness and disease and also affecting how quickly we recover when we get sick.

But, just like all other processes of ageing, immunosenescence doesn't just happen by itself. It is affected by diet and lifestyle, our stress levels, how much sleep we get, how we think and feel, and how we behave.

We have known for a long time that stress impacts the immune system. People under stress tend to get more colds and to be more prone to infections, for example.

Attitude affects the immune system, too. A generally positive attitude to life's stressors helps us to recover faster from everyday ailments.

But even though it's not something we consider in popular culture, the immune system also responds to displays and feelings of kindness, empathy, compassion, love, affection and elevation.

### The Mother Teresa effect

In a famous study by scientists at Harvard University, 132 students watched a 50-minute video of Mother Teresa performing acts of kindness. It was an inspiring video and they felt elevated by it.

Before and after the video, they had swabs taken of their saliva so that the scientists could measure the levels of an important component of their immune systems known as salivary immunoglobulin-A (s-IgA). It is the immune system's first line of defence against pathogens that we ingest in our food.

The scientists found that the students' s-IgA levels had increased significantly on watching the film. And not only that, but when they checked an hour later, the s-IgA levels were still high.

The scientists put the still elevated levels down to the students' elevation; they had 'continued to dwell on the loving relationships that characterized the film'.[20]

As within, so without... Elevation as we observe life on the outside elevates the immune system on the inside.

The results of this study are now affectionately known as the 'Mother Teresa effect'.

## ACT OF KINDNESS

*If you're getting a coffee for yourself in the office, offer to get one for your colleagues around you, or just surprise someone with a coffee on your return.*

In another experiment, scientists at the HeartMath Institute in Boulder, Colorado, measured s-IgA levels in a group of volunteers and then asked them to create and hold a feeling of care and compassion for five minutes. Immediately afterwards, they measured their s-IgA levels again.

Even though it was just a small time period, the volunteers' s-IgA levels had increased by 50 per cent, and not only that, they remained elevated for some time, taking around five hours in fact to come back to normal.[21]

This clearly shows that when we have feelings associated with kindness, care, compassion, elevation, love, affection and warm connection, our immune system gets a boost.

We benefit from the same kind of effect when someone shows us empathy. When a doctor, for instance, shows empathy, it relaxes us. It makes us feel listened to, comforted and hopeful, and this reduces much of the stress associated with seeing the doctor. It also makes all the difference to how the immune system responds and ultimately to how quickly we recover from illness.

This was shown in a randomized controlled trial of 719 patients with the common cold. Around half had a standard visit to their doctor and half had what was called an *enhanced* visit, where the doctor emphasized empathy. The patients filled out a CARE questionnaire (Consultation and Relational Empathy) afterwards so that the scientists could monitor empathy levels as perceived by the patients, which reflected how they felt during the consultation.

The duration of each patient's cold was measured, as well as their immune response. Those who had received an empathy-enhanced visit and given it a perfect score on the CARE questionnaire (223 patients), had a cold of reduced severity, recovered faster than everyone else and also had higher immune function. Just feeling cared for and listened to had a direct impact on their immune systems.[22]

What these three studies tell us is that we can boost our immune system through what we give our attention to and how we therefore feel.

Think about it the other way. Stress is often caused by what we focus on. A deadline at work can cause stress and the thought of the deadline can have the same effect. And this stress can suppress the immune system.

It's the same with kindness, except that the thoughts that bring about the feelings of kindness, connection, compassion and affection elevate the immune system instead.

# CHAPTER SUMMARY

❤ There are seven processes of ageing that can be slowed by kindness. They are: muscle degeneration, reduced vagal tone, inflammation, oxidative stress, depleted nitric oxide, shortened telomeres and immunosenescence.

❤ Kindness helps muscle regeneration because oxytocin plays a crucial role in the process. Without enough oxytocin, muscle regeneration is slower.

❤ Kindness also boosts vagal tone, enabling us to improve our ability to neutralize persistent (chronic) low-grade inflammation, which plays a role in many diseases and in ageing.

❤ In producing oxytocin, kindness is also able to help mop up the free radicals that cause oxidative stress. This is important for our arteries but also for the ageing of our tissues, particularly the skin. Free radicals play a key role in the formation of wrinkles. Thus, as we produce more oxytocin through kindness, we can slow the development of the more visible signs of ageing.

❤ Depleted nitric oxide is one of the most significant processes of ageing because nitric oxide is needed to maintain so many systems of the body. We can boost our nitric oxide through consistent thoughts, feelings and acts of kindness. Like oxytocin, nitric oxide is a molecule of kindness.

♥ Telomeres are the end caps on DNA. Slowing the wear and tear on them slows ageing, and kindness, compassion and emotional support have been shown to substantially slow the loss of telomere length.

♥ Immunosenescence is the gradual weakening of the immune system that occurs with age. The feelings of elevation that kindness produces, as shown in the Mother Teresa effect, can boost the immune system.

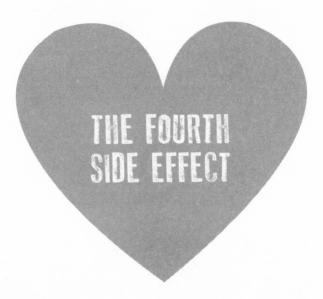

THE FOURTH
SIDE EFFECT

# Kindness Improves Relationships

*At the touch of love, everyone
becomes a poet.*

PLATO

'I pick kindness.'

That was the response given by a majority of people when asked what they most wanted in a prospective mate.

It was a large study of more than 10,000 young people aged 20–25, spanning 33 different countries across six continents. Without exception, right across the board in all these cultures, kindness was number one.[1]

This might come as a surprise. We might think that good looks or good financial prospects would be first. But that's because we typically think of how *other* people would respond. When asked what *we* want (and we take a moment or two to think about it), most of us pick kindness.

That's certainly the result I get time and time again when I do a straw poll at talks or workshops.

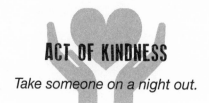

# ACT OF KINDNESS

*Take someone on a night out.*

## Survival of the Kindest

It's natural for us to be drawn to people who are kind. We find it attractive because some ancient instinct inside us knows that kindness is the foundation upon which all human life exists.

Let me take a moment to explain why we are drawn to kindness, so that we can come to understand how and why it improves relationships. It's all to do with our genes and how we evolved.

Our genes were shaped over millions of years. Here's how it works. Let's say one tribe of our ancient ancestors has gene A and the other has gene B. To make it little more colourful, let's say gene A is pink and gene B is blue.

Now the pink gene and the blue gene do very different things. The pink gene makes people share their resources and look out for one another's wellbeing. Think of it as a kindness gene. The blue gene, on the other hand, is very much a 'me first' gene, and people with this gene aren't that concerned about the wellbeing of others. As long as they're safe themselves, that's good enough.

Now, two processes work in nature to shape us. The first is about energy.

The pink gene tribe uses up less energy as a group because they share with one another, so only a few members of the tribe need to gather the food for the whole group. Gathering food costs the blue gene tribe much more energy as a group, because they're all fending for themselves.

Nature is quite efficient and tends to favour low-energy processes, because over time, as food availability fluctuates, the less energy we need to survive, the better. So the pink gene tribe thrives and grows much larger than the blue gene tribe. Eventually, in the overall gene pool, there are far more pink genes than blue genes.

## ACT OF KINDNESS

*Send chocolates at Christmas to a company that has provided you with a good service.*

The second natural process that shapes us is about forming bonds (relationships).

The pink gene tribe has strong relationships. The blue gene tribe has weak relationships. This is because the sharing in the pink gene tribe strengthens the relationships between its members.

You see the same kind of thing every day. People who share tend to develop good relationships, while people who are more selfish tend to have weaker relationships. It makes sense.

Coming back to the tribes again, the pink gene tribe thrives over a long period of time, because when there's danger from wild animals or other tribes, the people work together; when there's hunger, they share. The blue gene tribe don't. When there's hunger or danger, only a few survive.

This is known as 'survival of the fittest', but notice that the fittest isn't the biggest and strongest, which is how we tend to think about it, but the *kindest*. It's the pink gene tribe.

In a nutshell, kindness creates strong bonds between members of a group and gives the group strength. It's this strength that counts in the survival stakes. So, over time, there are many more pink genes than blue genes in the gene pool.

Now, winding the clock forward a few million years to the modern day, we *are* the pink gene tribe.

The pink gene is the oxytocin gene.[2] It's one of the oldest genes in the human genome, at a spritely 500 million years young.[3] Being so old, it has become integrated into a large number of our biological systems. This is *why* being kind affects us in so many beneficial ways: why it makes us happier, is good for our hearts and slows ageing.

Kindness has played a key role in the survival of the human species, not only in the ancient past but also in our modern world. Where would we be without kindness and cooperation?

Kindness creates relationships and strengthens existing ones. And it's the strength of our relationships that has got us to where we are today.

## The Little Things

*It's the little things that count. I was in a relationship with a man quite a few years ago. I'd liked him for some time and was thrilled when he asked me out. He was very handsome. I'd been single for a while and it was nice to be with someone again.*

*But being single had given me space to figure out what I wanted in a relationship. Being with a handsome man wasn't everything.*

*We'd been dating for a couple of months when one night, after going for a walk, we were sitting on a bench and I felt cold. I asked if I could borrow his jacket, but he wouldn't give it to me. He said he would be cold as he only had a shirt on underneath.*

*Don't get me wrong – he wasn't being unkind. He didn't say it in a mean way or anything like that. He just put himself first. That was all.*

*When I thought about it, I realized that that was how it had been from the start. He hadn't really done any of the little things, the important kind little things that make a person feel special or valued.*

*I decided that night that I didn't want to be in that relationship anymore and broke it off a few days later.*

*It's the little things that count, you see, as they all add up to be one big thing.*

HAZEL

## The Magic Ratio

John Gottman, Emeritus Professor of Psychology at the University of Washington, is famous for his work on relationships and marital stability. His work has in fact formed the basis for much of the marriage counselling movement.

By studying couples interacting with each other for just a short time, he is able to predict which relationships will stand the test of time. There's a magic ratio, he says, in how we relate to each other. So long as we say or do more than five positive things for one negative thing, the relationship is likely to work out. That's the magic ratio, 5:1.

Positives tend to include kindness, affection, love, support and listening; negatives tend to include contempt, hostility, anger, negative judgements, selfishness and indifference.

In one example of his work, Gottman and his colleagues studied 700 newlywed couples. The couples only spoke to each other for 15 minutes. Yet just by counting the positives and negatives, the psychologists predicted with 94 per cent accuracy who would still be together 10 years later.

# ACT OF KINDNESS

*Send flowers to an elderly person.*

Kindness is relationship glue. We don't really need science to tell us this – common sense and personal experience are our own laboratories, regardless of whether the relationship in question is with a loved one, a friend, a work colleague or a family member. But research like this is useful because it shines a light on some of the factors that are most important for building a lasting relationship.

In another piece of Gottman's work, he studied 130 newlywed couples going about a typical day. He described behaviour that we see every day in relationships, where one partner might for example request the other's attention with something along the lines of 'Come and see this.'

This is what he calls a 'bid'. It is simply a request for connection. It doesn't really matter what the person is drawing their partner's attention to; underneath, it's just the connection that they are seeking. The key is recognizing this and responding.

Gottman studied how people would respond to their partner's bid and found they would either 'turn toward' or 'turn away'.

Turning toward meant they basically gave their partner their attention – a display of kindness. Turning away, on the other hand, meant they didn't give their partner their attention, or that their response was half-hearted, like saying, 'Hmmm, yes, nice,' while keeping their focus trained on the TV or their phone, or that they even responded with contempt or hostility.

Gottman then followed up on the couples six years later. He found that those who were still together after this time had turned toward their partner 87 per cent of the time. Couples who had separated had only turned toward their partner 33 per cent of the time.[4]

A typical relationship sees bids for connection several times a day, each providing an opportunity for a little act of kindness. These may seem small and insignificant, but they are the glue that holds the relationship together.

In a romantic relationship, it's the little things that count because these make up the vast majority of the bids. The listening when you speak, the cups of tea, the back rubs, the helping with tasks, the responding to your needs, even after a day at work – these are the little kindnesses that count.

And as we offer these kindnesses, our relationship gets stronger and is more likely to stand the test of time.

In fact kindness is top of the list of factors that produce happiness and satisfaction in a relationship. This applies not only to our romantic relationships, but our relationships with friends, family members and work colleagues, too.

# ACT OF KINDNESS

*Visit an elderly person and
listen to their stories.*

## What's Your Style?

Another way we show kindness in a relationship is when our partner shares good news with us, giving us the opportunity to participate in it.

Shelly Gable, a psychology professor at the University of California Santa Barbara, has studied four kinds of response to the sharing of good news: active-constructive, passive-constructive, active-destructive and passive-destructive.

When one person tells their partner about something good that has happened to them, or gives other good news, if their partner responds with happiness or enthusiasm and is genuinely pleased, that is an *active-constructive* response.

A *passive-constructive* response is where a partner doesn't show a lot of interest, but the person knows they are interested really.

An *active-destructive* response is where a partner finds fault or focuses on potential negatives, essentially deflating their partner's happiness.

And a *passive-destructive* response is where a partner doesn't seem to care and the person knows they really aren't interested at all.

Gable enlisted 148 couples – 59 couples who had been dating for an average of a year and 89 couples who had been married for an average of 10 years. They were given the statement: 'When I tell my partner about something good that has happened to me…' and a series of responses that reflected each of the four types and asked to rate their responses on a scale from one to seven.

The results showed that how a partner responded made all the difference to the quality of the relationship and the chances of its survival. Commitment, trust, satisfaction and intimacy – measures of a good-quality relationship that is likely to last – were highest in couples whose responses were active-constructive. In other words, kindness, which is active-constructive responding, made for better relationships.[5]

(Please note, I've summarized each of the categories in just one sentence to give a general flavour of the styles, but there are more dimensions to each. Before labelling your own personal relationships, I'd encourage you to read the research yourself and explore the full dimensions of each style.)

## ACT OF KINDNESS

*Find out what a loved one or friend really wants and provide it for them.*

Gable then extended the study from couples to friends, siblings, parents and college roommates. This time she measured positive emotion and life satisfaction. She found that these too were higher when individuals were supported in an active-constructive way, regardless of whether it was by friends, siblings, parents or college roommates.[6]

Kindness from a friend or loved one makes us feel understood, validated, relevant. The reward when someone shows us kindness is that we like them better for it. Generally speaking, in any kind of relationship where there's kindness, there's more satisfaction, less conflict, less hostility, less anger and more fun and relaxation.

We all know, of course, that there's more to a relationship than just kindness, but kindness is the way to go if we want our relationships to last.

And although I'm talking a lot about kindness, we also know that love is central to a romantic relationship. Kindness is the route we take in expressing a lot of that love.

Given that kindness is what is really wanted, you don't have to be the most intelligent person to participate in a successful long-term relationship, nor do you have to be the funniest, nor the one with the best hair, the best body, the most prominent six-pack or the firmest muscle tone. The most important thing to be is kind. Listen. Be responsive. Watch out for bids and kindly engage in sharing whatever experience comes out of them.

Of course, you might argue that some people's bids for connection come from a sense of insecurity, resting on a shaky foundation of low self-esteem. That can be true. Bids like these are slightly different, though. They have less to do with connection and more to do with testing how much your partner loves you.

If you recognize this behaviour in yourself, you might benefit from building some healthy self-esteem. My book *I Heart Me: The Science of Self-Love* might be a good place to start, as it shares numerous practical strategies.

If you recognize this behaviour in your partner instead, ask yourself what would be a kind way to respond. We naturally resist such tests, but if we understand the insecurity behind them then we can initiate a conversation that can lead to working through insecurity and self-esteem.

## A Helping Hand

'I was nervous,' Elizabeth told me. She's an actress and it was an important audition for a big TV show. Big auditions can be overwhelming sometimes.

> *The casting director came to collect me, and as he was opening the door to show me into the room with the producers and director, he gave me praise for my performance in a short film that I'd also written and directed. I'd made it a year earlier and he told me he'd viewed it via the Scottish BAFTA entries.*

*'That's why you're here today, because of that
performance,' he said to me.*

*It was a really kind thing to do, as an audition for a big TV
show can be a nerve-racking thing. The casting director
understood that, as he used to be an actor himself.*

*His words gave me the confidence boost that I needed for
my audition and I felt that there was someone in the room
rooting for me. So much so that even though in the end I
wasn't right for the part, I gave such a good performance
that I was offered another part in a different episode off the
back of that audition.*

It's nice to be nice, as they say. A little bit of kindness can give someone the helping hand they need. Kindness brings out the best in people; it gives them the confidence and freedom to show their larger selves.

## ACT OF KINDNESS

*Buy a book for someone.*

Whatever our working environment, we work harder for people who are kind to us. We give our best performances, so to speak. Kindness creates a safety net for us. We feel it's okay to make mistakes. So we feel it's okay to stretch ourselves too, and quite often we stretch into a new version of ourselves.

*I had a really critical boss once. She was so critical of the tiniest detail that I felt nervous around her. So I kept making mistakes. And then she was really critical of me for making them. And the more critical she was, the more afraid I was of making mistakes and the more I kept making.*

*The thing is, I'd done so well with the manager I'd had before her. Joe had been really kind – such a lovely guy. He'd always been helpful and supportive, and so easy to approach when I wasn't sure of what I was doing. In fact he'd really believed in me. He'd give me extra challenges because he'd been sure that I could handle them.*

*I loved my job when Joe was in charge. But then he moved up in the company and the critical woman took over.*

*The difference one person can make! They were like night and day. Joe was kind. She wasn't. My performance dropped so much and I withdrew into my shell. I stopped enjoying my job. It was horrible really.*

*Eventually I applied for other jobs and was lucky enough to get another one within the company, thanks to a recommendation from Joe, as it happens.*

CLAIRE

Many of us can relate to Claire's experience. A boss who is kind, who sees the best in us, brings out the best in us. It's as if we have permission to be ourselves, to stretch ourselves in new directions, to try out new ways of being. Kindness expands us. Criticism, on the other hand, when it's given unkindly, makes us shrink. We're less likely to stretch ourselves in new directions because we fear being pulled up for any mistakes we make.

*In business, there can sometimes be a severe lack of compassion. It can be a dog-eat-dog world. There are decisions to be made based on financial outcomes and there's no room for heartfelt stuff. Or at least, that's what I thought until we hired a new recruit named Willie.*

*My job was in sales, and Willie and I had to bring in a certain amount of revenue every month or we'd be sacked. I was Willie's boss. I was doing okay, but he was struggling. To be honest, he wasn't the best salesman in the world, but he was a diamond of a man – rough, but worth his weight in gold.*

*Two months went by and our work was being evaluated the day before a board meeting to decide who was worth keeping. I was fine. Willie, on the other hand, was not. His sales figures were way down and according to company policy he should have been given the boot. But when it came to the board meeting, he was kept on. His sales figures had magically grown overnight.*

*I had a soft spot for Willie and I'd transferred some of my own sales onto his figures. I knew that he had a family to support and I didn't want him to be out of a job. No one knew this except me, not even Willie himself.*

*There is always room for compassion in business, you just have to look for the opportunity.*

PETER

Peter told me that he helped Willie a lot over the following years and Willie helped him, too. Willie appreciated that Peter was someone he could always go to for guidance and support, and they became lasting friends.

Andy told me another story about kindness in business:

*There was this guy who worked for me. His name was Gary. He helped me a lot when I first joined the company, although I was much more senior than him.*

*He worked as a technician, but he could do just about anything. Whenever I had a problem, he was the first person I'd ask. He knew how all the instruments worked and he was also a nice guy, always willing to put what he was doing aside when someone asked for help.*

*Before long, I grew to learn how things worked in the company. There were certain barriers. A technician without a university degree could never progress beyond grade 9, yet the entry level of a university graduate was grade 11. That was the rule.*

*I didn't think that was fair. Gary was very intelligent and could easily have done a graduate's job. So one day I went to the head of department and told him how helpful*

*Gary had been to me since I'd joined the company. The department head was a nice person and he respected me a lot. I told him these barriers were discouraging to people and that we needed to allow exceptions, and these exceptions might encourage others to stretch themselves, which could only be good for the company.*

*He thought about it for a few days, then he dropped into my office one morning to say he would like to offer Gary a promotion. Gary would become the first person in the department without a degree to be promoted to a graduate-level position. I was thrilled for him.*

*The department head also told Gary that I'd fought his corner for him, which I thought was a nice thing to do, because I wasn't going to say anything about it.*

*Gary was so grateful. We've been friends for 20 years now.*

ANDY

## Looking Out for Little Sister

*I was due to go to a party and was so looking forward to it. I don't exactly get out that much, as I am a single mum. But then I got a call from my babysitter: she wasn't well and couldn't come.*

*Shortly afterwards, a friend who had arranged to pick me up in her car knocked on my door, dressed up to the nines, only to meet an exasperated and underdressed woman with two kids on her hands.*

*I told her just to go on and enjoy herself, but she was having none of it. She flew into action and called up every previous babysitter that I'd ever used. She found one who was free and then told me to get dressed – quickly! – while she got the kids ready to go in her car.*

*Moments later, we were on our way to the babysitter's. We dropped the kids off and arrived at the restaurant where all our colleagues were waiting just an hour late.*

*My friend could easily have left me at the house and got to the dinner on time, but she didn't. My happiness was important to her and she sacrificed some of her evening for me. Kindness to a tee. A friend for life!*

CAROLYN

Kindness is the glue that holds friendships together, too. Carolyn would certainly agree.

Kindness deepens a friendship, whether we're there for a friend in need or we're the one in need and a friend is there for us.

With a new friendship, kindness helps cement the bond, removing emotional distance in the early stages and making it easier to relate to the other person.

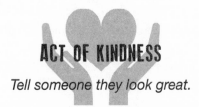

# ACT OF KINDNESS

*Tell someone they look great.*

During a gift-giving week known as 'Big Sister Week', older members of the sorority at the University of Virginia give gifts to new members as a way of welcoming them and bringing them into the fold of the larger group.

During a Big Sister Week that was studied by psychologists at the university, 78 'big sisters' organized gifts to be delivered to 82 'little sisters', organized events for them and ensured that they were pampered throughout the week. It was all done anonymously until the end of the week, when the big sisters revealed their identities.

At the end of the week and again one month later, psychologists from the university asked the little sisters to tell them about the benefits they had received during the week and asked both big sisters and little sisters to report on their relationships after the week ended.

They found, perhaps unsurprisingly, that the big sisters had forged friendships with the little sisters and that the kindness of the big sisters was an important factor in these new relationships. But also important was the gratitude of the little sisters. In a sense, this gratitude was a reciprocal kindness, because it rested on a wish to repay the kindness of the big sisters. The little sisters who felt the most gratitude were in fact enjoying the best relationships with the big sisters. They also felt more integrated into the sorority.[7]

# ACT OF KINDNESS

*Buy a large box of cakes and pastries and give them out on the street.*

Gratitude is especially important in our relationships with our friends and loved ones because time causes us to forget much of the good they have brought into our lives. Seeing a person every day and getting caught up in the challenges and circumstances of life causes us to forget how important they are to us. Unfortunately, many of us only remember when it is too late. The divorce courts are littered with the corpses of relationships where one person took the other for granted.

Gratitude encourages us to notice the blessings in both our romantic relationships and our friendships. We start to recall things that we've forgotten that were significant at an earlier time. And so we start to show more kindness towards our partners and friends.

Kindness begets gratitude and gratitude begets kindness. It's a circle.

# ACT OF KINDNESS

*Throw a party for someone who
deserves some appreciation.*

## Kindness Breaks Through

*We visited a dog rescue centre some years ago. There was
this one dog sitting at the back of a cage that had several
other dogs in it. She had her head down and was facing the
corner. We just knew right away that she was our girl. We
needed to give her a forever home.*

*Her name was Ariel. When we brought her home, she was
so very shy and nervous that I'm sure she must have been
badly treated in her last home. She wouldn't come to us
at first. But we just kept showing her kindness. I'd slowly
move beside her and gently rub her head, and she'd lie
there and let me do it.*

*Gradually she became more responsive. It's funny, but
I remember the little things the most. I remember the
first time she wagged her tail when she saw me coming
towards her. She knew that I would rub her head. Her
tail just began to move a little, a slow beat on the carpet,
up and down, up and down. It was the sweetest thing. It
made me want to cry.*

*We just kept showing her love. We spoke kindly to her and gave her lots of nice treats. Before long she had completely settled in and become one of the family.*

*Dogs don't ask for much. If you're kind to them, you'll have a friend for life.*

DENISE

Kindness not only strengthens human relationships, but strengthens relationships with animals, too. Kindness is kindness is kindness. It's all the same.

## ACT OF KINDNESS

*Offer to tidy an elderly neighbour's garden.*

There was a time several years ago when we had a large fish tank in our office. One day as my friend Kenny and I passed the room with the tank in, we saw that one of the office girls was kneeling down with her eyes closed and her hands cupped against the tank. Kenny asked what she was doing.

She looked up and said, 'The little fish is sick. I'm praying for it.'

Kenny just looked at me, nodded and said, 'Yup! She knows what it's all about.'

# CHAPTER SUMMARY

❤ Kindness is what most of us want in a partner. It's what we find most attractive and what people find attractive in us.

❤ Our ancient ancestors learned that it was easier to share and that there was safety in numbers. This is why kindness is our nature. It's also why it's so healthy for us. The gene that produces oxytocin is over 500 million years old and has become integrated into a large number of our body's systems, which means these systems respond to kindness. That's *why* kindness makes us happier, is good for our heart and slows ageing.

❤ Kindness helps us shine. It helps us be the best we can be. We always remember the acts of kindness that helped us to expand.

❤ Kindness is also what makes friendships and relationships successful. Our friends and loved ones make bids for connection several times a day and when we respond actively and supportively, it increases the chances of our relationships standing the test of time.

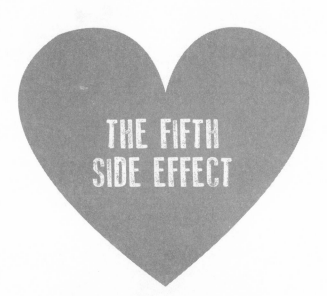

# THE FIFTH SIDE EFFECT

# Kindness Is Contagious

*Remember there's no such thing as a small act of kindness. Every act creates a ripple with no logical end.*

Scott Adams

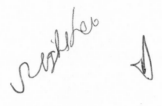

**Contagious [kuh n-tey-juh s]**: Capable of being transmitted from one person or organism to another.

I was sitting in a coffee shop when I saw a young girl. She was probably about 19 or 20, I guess. She walked past a homeless man, paused for a second, then walked on.

She reappeared a few minutes later carrying a brown bag with some food and what I assume was a hot drink. She handed it to the man and they spoke for a few minutes. Then she walked away.

It was a beautiful act of kindness, unnoticed by most of the world, and most likely the girl won't say anything to anyone either. But it really touched me. I felt uplifted, inspired even.

When I left the coffee shop about an hour or so later, I found myself stopping to hand £10 to a homeless person. Usually I'd just hand £1 or some change. For the rest of the day I found myself making an extra effort to be helpful to people – family, friends, shop assistants – not just helping them, but giving them my full attention when they spoke and responding in ways that I thought would make them feel good about themselves.

When I went to bed that night, I reflected on the day. Wasn't it amazing, I thought, how the young girl's act of kindness towards the homeless man had had a larger effect?

Her kindness had actually *caused* the other homeless man to receive £10, shop assistants to exchange some smiles and my family and friends to receive help and support. Through one simple act of kindness, she had set in motion a chain of positive events.

This kind of thing happens every day. We just don't notice it.

Just as a pebble dropped in a pond creates ripples that lift lily pads on the other side, so acts of kindness lift the spirits of people who witness it and they carry that kindness forward, lifting the spirits of others.

This is called a ripple effect, or domino effect.

##  The Source of a Ripple Effect

*Please think of a specific time when you saw someone demonstrate humanity's higher or better nature … [where] you saw someone doing something good, honourable, or charitable for someone else [or] please think of a specific time when someone did something really good for you.*

These were the instructions given by psychologists Sarah Algoe and Jonathan Haidt to 162 students who participated in a kindness study.

Afterwards, the students were asked to describe their physical sensations, motivation and any actions they took. Those who had witnessed kindness reported a warm feeling in the chest and a desire to emulate the kindness they saw. Those who had kindness shown to them felt gratitude and a desire to repay the kindness and were motivated to emulate that kind behaviour.[1]

The research seems to show that it is elevation that is the source of kindness ripple effects. Jonathan Haidt describes it in the following way: 'Elevation is elicited by acts of moral beauty; it causes warm, open feelings in the chest; and it motivates people to behave more virtuously themselves.'[2]

When we witness kindness, we feel uplifted. We often have warm, expansive sensations in our chest area – in our heart.

'It makes me want to hug the world,' as a friend said.

Indeed, in the next part of their study, Algoe and Haidt asked 114 students to make a note of kindnesses they witnessed over the next three weeks. Afterwards, they reported that they wanted to 'do something good for another', 'be like the other person' and 'be a better person'.

# ACT OF KINDNESS

*Send a card to one of your old schoolteachers or university professors and tell them how much they influenced your life.*

As a 22-month-old child, Joel Sonnenberg was badly burned and disfigured after a tractor trailer hit the family's car. He lost his toes, his fingers and one hand. He also had to go through 45 operations over the next few years as surgeons did their best to aid his recovery.

At first the driver, Mr Dort, said his brakes had failed, but it later turned out that he had actually been trying to hit a female acquaintance. Joel's pain and disfigurement had been the result of an aggressive act that was intended to harm.

In a study led by scientists at the University of Delaware and the University of British Columbia, volunteers were shown a video of Joel's story plus segments of the sentencing hearing.

In the video, Joel's mother said, 'I do forgive you, Mr Dort. You will see my scarred Joel this morning. All of us have scars.'

Joel's father offered, 'When you ask my forgiveness, I will forgive you.'

When Joel himself spoke, he said, 'This is my prayer for you: that you may know that grace has no limits. We will not consume our lives with hatred, because hatred brings only misery. We will surround our lives with love.' ⫻

When they finished watching the video, the volunteers were asked how they felt.

Elevated! They felt uplifted by the grace, compassion and forgiveness that Joel and his family had shown towards the tractor driver who had had such a terrible impact on their lives. And it motivated all of them to become better people.[3]

Elevation uplifts us and produces an immediate desire to emulate the kindness we witness. It inspires us to carry the spirit of kindness forward.

## One Kind Act Leads to Another

Motivation usually leads to action. Elevation motivates us to be kind, so we will follow through with actual kindnesses.

Sometimes we plan them – we think of helping particular people in our lives and then we act. Sometimes we simply act on opportunities as they present themselves.

### ACT OF KINDNESS

*When a new person joins the company you work for or moves into your street, make them feel welcome by taking them for lunch.*

In one piece of research that examined how elevation actually motivated kindness, one group of volunteers was shown a morally uplifting video clip and another group was shown a funny clip (for comparison purposes). The uplifting clip was from *The Oprah Winfrey Show*.

The volunteers who watched the uplifting clip reported feeling uplifted, optimistic about humanity, warm in the chest and/or happy, as we might have expected.

But the key to the experiment was the next part. Did the effect stop at motivation or did people actually follow through?

The volunteers were asked to help with a different task. Would those who felt elevated after witnessing kindness be more likely to help than those who had merely had a laugh? Indeed they were. Those who had watched the Oprah clip were the ones most likely to help.[4]

And in a separate experiment, the researchers found that those who had experienced elevation after watching the Oprah clip actually spent twice as long helping them with a task as those who had watched the comedy clip.[5]

I've found that when I recall witnessing kind acts, or when I think of times when I've received help when I really needed it, I feel uplifted. It makes me feel happy sometimes for hours afterwards. It's a very useful self-help exercise for improving your mood.

It has to be done *on purpose*, though. What I mean here is that there's a difference between the mind drifting towards happy memories and choosing to think of happy memories. The latter is an intervention: you're intending to feel better and you're using the happy memories as a tool to do that. And that makes all the difference.

I've noticed that when I do this, I often remember to do kind things that I'd intended to do but just not got around to doing.

I also find that when I practise the loving-kindness meditation I feel more compassionate for a while afterwards and also more likely to follow through on helpful things that I hadn't got around to doing.

In an online loving-kindness meditation study, 809 people were randomized to do the loving-kindness meditation or take a light physical exercise course. Afterwards they were given the option of donating half of their study payment to charity. More of those who did the meditation donated money than those who did the light exercise.[6]

## Child-sized Ripples

Psychologists Harriet Over and Malinda Carpenter showed 60 18-month-old infants some photographs of household objects, for example a teapot. In the background of the photo were two wooden dolls.

How the dolls were positioned was the key to the experiment. Some of the infants were shown the two dolls standing very close together and facing each other, depicting love or togetherness, some were shown the dolls with their backs to one another or just a single doll, and one group saw a neutral stack of blocks instead of dolls. The scientists wanted to see if the positioning of the dolls would influence the infants' behaviour.

Each child would play with the experimenter and an assistant for a while, then would look at the photos. Immediately afterwards, the experimenter would leave the room and return with a bundle of pencils which she would then 'accidentally' drop. What the researchers wanted to see was which children helped pick up the pencils.

It turned out that 60 per cent of the children who had seen the dolls facing each other in the photos spontaneously (within 10 seconds) helped pick up the pencils, yet only 20 per cent of the children in the other groups helped. This means that after seeing a photo depicting love, the infants were three times more likely to show kind behaviour than if they were shown a different orientation of dolls.[7]

This is a very important phenomenon because it shows just how sensitive children are to what they see around them. When we display kindness, or even just depict love or kindness in some way, it impacts how infants and children behave.

In a more direct study, children watched a video of people bowling, but one group witnessed the winner give his winning certificate to charity whereas the other group were not shown this part.

Later, when all of the children were given certificates themselves, those who saw the full video were more likely to give their certificates away than the group who didn't see that part.[8]

In another study, children watched a Lassie movie, again with two endings. Lassie movies were very famous in the 1970s. I remember being glued to the TV when I was a child, watching Lassie, a collie dog, show extraordinary courage and compassion.

In the movie that the children watched, some of them witnessed Lassie's owner rescue her puppies, but others weren't shown this part. Afterwards, all of the children played a points-scoring game that was interrupted by the sounds of distressed puppies. Even though they would lose points in the game if they left, the children who saw the puppies being rescued in the Lassie movie were more likely than the others to go and help.[9]

Children are also easily influenced by other children being kind. Researchers at Arizona State University studied the interactions of 124 boys and girls throughout a school term with the help of their teachers, who were asked to keep a note of when children showed helpfulness and what they did.

The following term the children were monitored again and it was found that the children who played with children who were deemed to be 'prosocial' (i.e. helpful, kind) experienced more positive emotion and less negative emotion. The researchers pointed out that this increase in positive emotion made it more likely that these children would become more prosocial themselves. In other words, children hanging out with children who are kind become kinder themselves.[10]

# ACT OF KINDNESS

*Buy some pet food and put it in an animal
charity collection bin in the supermarket.*

Most parents worry about the opposite happening: that their
children are associating with others who are a bad influence. This
can happen. Once when I was a child and found myself associating
with a group who regularly got into trouble, one declared to me, 'If
you fly with the crows, you get caught with the crows.'

The one and only time I ever stole something was around this
time. I remember being instructed on an 'easy' theft, as my friend
called it. It was close to 5 November, the annual Guy Fawkes
Day. We went into a shop and shoved some fireworks up the
sleeves of our coats before walking back out. This was in the
days before CCTV cameras. I remember feeling physically sick
afterwards, not from the fear of getting caught, but from the guilt
of having stolen something. I vowed never to do anything like
that again and I knew that I could no longer hang around with
those boys.

But, just as some children can be bad influences, others are
good influences. I was lucky enough to gradually make friends
who were very different and had good, strong values that were
rooted in honesty and kindness.

Later, when I went to university, my friend Stuart had an impact
on me. I remember feeling elevated by the way he was always

there for his friends, always offering help when someone needed it. He once shared one of his guiding principles, which he'd learned from his mum: 'If you don't have anything nice to say then don't say anything at all.' It has stuck with me to this day and still forms part of my philosophy of life.

Incidentally, Stuart was one of the most liked people at university.

## Contagious Kindness in the Workplace

'When my head of department is nice, I'm more helpful to my subordinates too,' explained Victoria.

Of course kindness ripples happen at work too. When a manager is kind and respectful towards their employees, the employees enjoy their jobs more and actually do a better job too.

Most of us have had this experience. In my time working in the pharmaceutical industry, I did my best work while having an immediate manager who was helpful and approachable and would go that extra mile to ensure that I enjoyed my job and had the support I needed.

This was echoed in a study led by Richard Netemeyer at the McIntyre School of Commerce at the University of Virginia, which assessed the performance and job satisfaction of 306 store managers in a women's clothing and accessories retail chain.

It also measured the job satisfaction levels and performance of 1,615 frontline staff and the customer satisfaction levels of 57,656 customers.

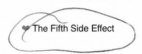

It found that the satisfaction levels of the managers caused a ripple effect. They impacted how the frontline employees felt and therefore how they did their job, which then cascaded down to how satisfied the customers felt on each visit to the store. In fact, using a seven-point scale of job satisfaction, each single point increase in a manager's satisfaction rippled through to a 5 per cent increase in customer spending, which amounted to each customer spending on average US$3.64 extra on every visit to the store.[11]

Happy employees treat customers better, and the kinder, more helpful, respectful and supportive a manager is, the happier an employee is likely to be. And that happiness and spirit of helpfulness usually ripples out to other people they interact with in the company.

## ACT OF KINDNESS

*Hold a door open for someone.*

A study led by Joseph Chancellor at the University of California, Riverside, found evidence that kindness spread in the workplace. Participants were randomized to be either Givers (those performing acts of kindness), Receivers (those receiving acts of kindness) or controls (neither giving nor receiving).

The study found a few things. First, that the Givers and Receivers both became happier, but also that the Receivers chose to do acts of kindness themselves in a 'pay-it-forward' fashion.[12] The kindness was contagious.

Another study showed that when a boss was kind, polite, fair, respectful and even self-sacrificing, employees tended to feel elevation and this made contagious kindness likely. It also created more positive attitudes, better relationships and a stronger commitment to the organization.

The study enlisted 121 volunteers in a medium-sized Italian company that supplied residential wooden doors and had an annual budget of around 25 million euros. The researchers created a fictitious leader, Massimo Castelli, who demonstrated inspiring interpersonal fairness and self-sacrifice.

They found that those who believed that Massimo Castelli treated his employees with 'politeness, respect and sensibility' and 'made sacrifices himself in order to help the company' reported feeling warmth in their chests and relaxed muscles (the physical sensations of elevation), a desire to be a better person and a desire to do something good for others.[13]

Kindness uplifts the human spirit in any environment and usually results in further kindness. And in a work environment it means happier customers, too.

## ACT OF KINDNESS

*Write and send a thank-you card
to a company that has provided
you with a good service.*

## Counting the Dominoes

James Fowler, a medical geneticist and social scientist at UC San Diego, and Nicholas Christakis, a former professor at Harvard but now professor of social and natural sciences at Yale, have done a lot of research on ripple effects.

They have shown that emotions are contagious through social networks, where one person feeling happier causes those around them to feel happier, who cause those around them to feel happier, and so on.[14] They have done the same kind of thing with kindness, and in a first of its kind scientific study they measured how far the ripples of kindness went.

To accomplish this, they made use of a game that's used in experimental economics known as the 'Public Goods Game'. In the game, players are invited to invest in the public good, a pot of money that is then multiplied and the result shared. The players get to keep what they have at the end of the game, so what often happens is that some people invest more and some people invest less. Larger investments are usually considered prosocial, in that they are generally intended to benefit everyone.

Usually the contributions are secret, but Fowler and Christakis allowed participants to see what others contributed. They wanted to measure what happened when someone made a larger than average contribution to the public good pot; in other words, when someone showed extra kindness.

Several rounds of the game were played, with the participants changed each time, so that each person in a game played the next round with different players.

They found that when one person made a much larger contribution, the other players in that game then made a larger than average contribution in the next game *they* played. The kind act of one person inspired the others to follow suit. But it didn't stop there. It rippled out over subsequent games.

Fowler and Christakis calculated that the ripple effect extended to three degrees of separation, that is, through three further rounds after the first larger donation.[15]

This in fact points towards what happens in real life. Ordinary acts of kindness spread beyond the actual person helped.

In real life, the 'three-degree rule' means that each time we are kind, we inspire someone else to be kind (one degree), who inspires someone else (two degrees), who inspires someone else (three degrees). And of course in real life we inspire more than one person at a time, and each of these also inspires further people, which is what Fowler and Christakis also showed.

On average, if your kind act inspires four people, and each of them does something kind that inspires four more people, who each inspire four more, then just from your single act of kindness you will have indirectly helped 64 people (4 × 4 × 4). And most of them you will never meet in your lifetime.

In other words, in any one day you're likely to be touching the lives of dozens or even hundreds of people without realizing, just as a single pebble dropped in a pond will lift dozens or even hundreds of lily pads on the surface of the water.

## ACT OF KINDNESS

*Slip some money into the purse or
pocket of someone who needs it,
so that when they find it they think
they must have misplaced it.*

## The World's Longest Kidney Donor Chain

On 26 March 2015, 77-year-old Mitzi Neyens of Wausau, Wisconsin, received a kidney from Matt Crane, of Philadelphia, whose wife, Michelle, had received a kidney from another donor.

Mitzi was the final link in a donor chain of 34 consecutive transplants initiated by a single altruistic donor, which had involved 26 different hospitals and stretched the length and breadth of the USA over the previous three months. It was the world's longest ever kidney donor chain.[16]

A kidney donor chain happens when someone receives a kidney and a family member or close friend then donates one of theirs to someone in need. None of them happen to be a biological match for their loved one, so they make a 'pay-it-forward' commitment instead.

Either a family member or a friend of the recipient of that kidney then does the same thing, pledging their kidney to someone else. And a family member or friend of that recipient does the same, and so on, until the chain breaks through illness or for some other reason.

Kathy Hart, an attorney from Minneapolis, was the altruistic donor who started Mitzi's chain. She got the idea because she heard a yoga instructor's son needed a kidney but she didn't think she would be a match, so she decided to join the National Kidney Register[17] and offer a kidney to someone who was a match. Peggy Hansmann, of Plymouth, Wisconsin, received her kidney.

The National Kidney Registry (NKR) was founded by Jan and Garet Hil after their 10-year-old daughter was suddenly diagnosed with kidney failure. None of the family were biologically compatible and they only found a donor after several unsuccessful attempts. A kidney was eventually donated by their daughter's 23-year-old-cousin on 12 July 2007.

The Hils founded the NKR with a mission to 'Save and improve the lives of people facing kidney failure by increasing the quality, speed, and number of living donor transplants in the world' and a vision that 'Every incompatible or poorly compatible living donor in the world will pass through a common registry and find a well-matched living donor in under six months.' So the organization was set up in the spirit of kindness, to spare families the possibility of losing their loved ones by not being able to find a match quickly enough.

Garet Hil himself donated one of his kidneys as part of the NKR's first kidney paired exchange programme. Eight people received a kidney from the chain that began with his donation.

## ACT OF KINDNESS

*Give someone a hug for no reason.*

A kidney donor chain is really quite extraordinary and contains countless amounts of care, compassion and kindness. It's not just the donors and recipients who are involved – each operation requires a team of surgeons, nurses and support staff. There are also the teams who transport the kidneys from one hospital to the next, linking several hospitals in several towns, all with a common purpose and all experiencing elevation as a result of the extraordinary acts of kindness they witness.

Each donor chain saves many lives, but it also elevates countless people who become part of it, from the donors and recipients themselves to the families and close friends who live in the knowledge that a single kind act started a chain that saved their loved one's life.

## Full Circle

Kindness very often comes full circle. Think about it in this simple way. If you do something kind that improves your environment, you have to live in that environment, so you benefit from it. I once shared that idea with a friend, who replied, 'Like if I take a leak in a swimming pool, I have to swim in the water?'

Kind of!

But in a real way, you're likely to be familiar with the idea that 'what goes around comes around' or 'you get back what you give out'. People tend to help those who help others, so kindness does very often come back to bless you.

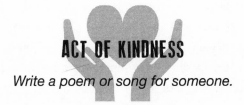

## ACT OF KINDNESS

*Write a poem or song for someone.*

While on a hike on a warm day, a young man by the name of Howard Kelly knocked on the door of a farmhouse and asked if he could possibly have a glass of water. A young girl answered and, wishing to show him some extra kindness, offered him a glass of milk instead. He was very grateful for it.

Years later he became a distinguished doctor. One day he discovered that the girl who had given him the glass of milk was receiving treatment at the hospital at which he worked.

Realizing that she was unlikely to be able to afford the high charges for her medical care, he obtained her bill, wrote upon it in bold handwriting, 'Paid in full with one glass of milk' and signed it.

Dr Howard Kelly was well known for his many kindnesses and was one of four founders of John Hopkins, which was the first medical research university in the USA. He was known to charge high rates for his services, but he used much of the income from these to fund treatments for patients who couldn't afford their care.[18]

## Spread the Word

Kindness ripples! There's no question about it. And one of the ways each of us can help the process along is to talk about the kind things we've witnessed, done or been on the receiving end of. Set up kindness discussion groups and share your experiences with others. Share videos through social media. The more people who are elevated by witnessing or learning about acts of kindness, the more kindness ripples we create.

### ACT OF KINDNESS

*Search out inspirational or funny videos on YouTube, Facebook or any other social media outlet, or other inspirational or funny material, and send it to someone who needs it.*

Here's a story to get you started.

Several years ago, I was working in the office of a charity that some friends and I had set up.[19] Most of us had put so many of our own resources into it that we ended up broke.

There was a time when I was really struggling, wondering how I was going to afford the week's bus fare to the office, when I received an envelope in the post. It contained £20 and a note that simply said, 'God bless!' I felt moved to tears by this heartfelt act of kindness. It was like a lottery win to me. I had an inkling about who might have sent it but I never said anything to them. I thought they'd prefer to remain anonymous.

Little did they know that their act of kindness would one day be written about in a book and touch the hearts of thousands of people!

A pebble dropped in a pond will always create ripples. An act of kindness will always do the same.

I try to be kind, but I didn't suddenly wake up one day and decide that kindness was important – I learned it. As I mentioned earlier, my mum has been a great example to me. Most of us can relate to this. We all learn from other people. So why not be an example of kindness and let others learn from you?

> *I was in my car going to collect my elderly friend Dorothy. On the way I reached the bottom of a steep hill and saw a guy struggling up it carrying a large TV.*
>
> *I stopped and offered him a lift. He was extremely grateful to me. We both lifted the TV into the car and I drove him over the hill to the other side. We took the TV out of the car and he offered me some money for helping him. I think he might have thought I was a taxi driver.*

*I refused, but he was insistent, so I made a deal with him. I said, 'Instead of giving me money, do something kind for someone. Pay it forward.'*

*He thought this was a good idea. We said our goodbyes and I drove on to collect Dorothy.*

*We were driving back about 10 minutes later when we saw the same man carrying the TV back over the hill.*

*I pulled up alongside him and asked him what he was doing. He said, 'I'm taking the damn thing back!'*

*He had stolen the TV.*

Tom

Tom's story makes me laugh because he said the guy was genuinely annoyed at the fact that he was taking the TV back, but knew it was the right thing to do. Clearly he had been inspired.

There are so many stories of kindness that I could tell you. Here are some more.

*Recently I was in the Outlet Store in Tillicoultry. [It's a village in central Scotland not far from Stirling.]*

*I picked up a small umbrella and a tablecloth, which I wanted to give as a present. I paid for the tablecloth, but realized when I got home that I hadn't paid for the umbrella. I didn't want to trail back to the store, so I just posted off a cheque for the money, not expecting to hear anymore about it.*

*Two weeks later I got a phone call from the store manager. He was completely astounded that I'd sent a cheque. He apologized for the lack of vigilance in the store, thanked me for my honesty and returned my cheque to me! Howzat!*

Jo

Elizabeth and I were moving house a few years ago. We didn't actually have that far to go. It was just down the road, so we didn't bother with a van or a removals company. But after filling our car with boxes and stuff for about the 10th time, driving it down the road, emptying it and carrying all the stuff up a flight of stairs, we realized that we hadn't really thought it through.

We started at 7:30 a.m. and by 5 p.m. there were only our two sofas left to move. The day before we'd decided that we could easily carry them down the road. It didn't seem quite such a good idea now.

So there we were, carrying the first sofa and stopping every 10 metres for a rest. It was especially hard for Elizabeth, as she is half my size. We'd got about 50 metres when a man who was walking along the road stopped, introduced himself as Tony and offered some help. It turned out that he would be one of our neighbours in the apartment complex we were moving to. So Tony and I carried the sofa down the rest of the road. It might not have seemed like much to him, but it made a huge difference to us.

But we were only half done. We still had another sofa, albeit a smaller two-seater, to take to the new apartment. So about

15 minutes later, it was *déjà vu* as we were carrying it down the road and stopping every 10 metres or so for a short rest.

This time we'd got about 80 metres down the road when a white van stopped and two Polish men jumped out. They didn't speak any English, but with a few friendly gestures they picked up the sofa. We all carried it down the road together, exchanging nods and smiles. Elizabeth held open the doors in the apartment complex as we squeezed the sofa around corners and up the stairs. The Polish men carried it all the way into the lounge without a word. When they placed it down, they just smiled and nodded again, then walked out of the door.

We were so grateful we felt moved to tears. I've never forgotten that.

## ACT OF KINDNESS

*If someone does something kind for you, do something kind for someone else. Pay it forward.*

*Today, my sister and I saw an older amputee woman begging on the ground on Princes Street in Edinburgh.*

*As we got closer to her, we saw she was feeding a pigeon, breaking up bread so the bird could eat. Even though she appeared to have very little, she was taking care of the beings around her.*

*That really moved us and we stopped and gave her some
money. She held our hands and told us she loved us. We
told her we loved her, too. I don't know if I've ever seen
eyes like hers, full of so much love that they absolutely
sparkled. It was a really special moment, human to human.*

Ems[20]

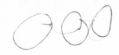

## A Chink of Light

A few years ago my friend Kim and her husband, Sinclair, were
struck by the terrible tragedy of losing their son, Calum, to
meningitis.

'I've never known darker days,' Kim said. 'The world was a very
bleak place for me at that time. I lost my love of life as well as
my son.'

It was every parent's worst nightmare. But the kindness of family,
friends and even strangers brought them hope. They received
lots of kind and heartfelt wishes, and friends visited and made
tea, did shopping, offered support and helped in any way they
could. Letters arrived from people they didn't know. They even
had hugs from neighbours they'd only ever said 'hello' to in the
past.

*The kindness spread around the world as people heard of
our fundraising efforts in aid of research into meningitis.
The band The Fratellis (Calum's favourite) gave us not only
a treasured guitar, a painting and a drum skin, but also their*

*time. They arranged to get my car out of the pound after it got towed away when I went to see them, asked to meet my son's friends, promoted the work of the Meningitis Trust and dedicated their album to Calum. So many other people helped raise funds and wished us well, too.*

A man from the United States entered a competition to win Fratellis merchandise so that he could send it to Kim and Sinclair to help their fundraising. A woman in England even sent them some of her personal collection of Fratellis goodies.

*These acts of kindness found a way to reach through the veil of tremendous grief and sadness. They created a chink of light that helped me to get through each day and begin to feel that the world wasn't a bad place. I'd never before been on the receiving end of such an outpouring of love and kindness.*

*The people who took the time to write, or bake, or shop or clean for us are our heroes. The friends who asked how we were and genuinely wanted to know, the ones who listened on the other end of the phone to my sobs at all hours can never be thanked enough. I know they didn't do any of these things to be thanked. But it is important for people to know the impact that their kind acts had.*

*These acts were fuel that helped to relight the fire within my soul. They touched a place deep within me that restored my faith in the world. This isn't to be taken lightly, as Calum's death made me question everything I'd previously believed in.*

*I doubt if the woman who baked some cakes and left them on our doorstep would have realized the impact that this had.*

*Kindness is so powerful. If everyone undertook the task of doing one act of kindness a week, think of how much light that could bring into the world.*

KIM

# CLOSING THOUGHTS

Every act of kindness matters. It matters to the people we help.

It also has side effects. We've learned that kindness makes us happier, benefits the heart, slows ageing, improves our relationships and is contagious.

Some argue that being kind is selfish if we know that we benefit from it. This issue will always be present. But we must not let the debate dissuade us from being kind. Regardless of any reasons, kindness makes a difference.

And in the moment of kindness, something takes over. It's the spirit of kindness. It warms our hearts and minds. It lifts us.

Kindness is bigger than our reasons for being kind. It's bigger than our debates, bigger than our philosophies, bigger even than our religions. Kindness is universal.

As Mark Twain wrote, 'Kindness is the language that the deaf can hear and the blind can see.'

Kindness connects us. It also ignites ancient biology that ensures the connection is a healthy one. There's a rightness to kindness.

Just as the act of dropping a pebble in water creates ripples, so an act of kindness ripples outwards, and in our modern interconnected world, it may impact many more people than we are aware of.

I read about a person recently who regularly stopped to buy coffee on his way to work. He would also buy coffee and a sandwich for a homeless man he passed on the street. Usually he'd pay for a few coffees in advance so that the man could drop into the shop during the day and have a warm drink.

One morning as he went into the coffee shop to buy the usual coffee and sandwich, the assistant told him that his coffee had already been paid for.

The homeless man – Daniel – had won £20 on a lottery scratchcard and one of the first things he'd done with it was pay for the coffee of the man who always paid for his.[1]

It's these seemingly little things – the small exchanges, the smiles, the helping hands – that make the difference in our world. They warm the heart. In this way, kindness forms the fabric of human society. It holds our families, friendships and communities together.

Kindness also lifts the spirit. It elevates us. It reminds us of who we are and what life is all about.

If ever you're in doubt as to what to do or in which direction to turn, be kind. For kindness is *always* the right thing, and it's always the right way.

# THE SEVEN-DAY
# KINDNESS CHALLENGE

I'd like to challenge you to perform at least one act of kindness a day for seven days in a row. The intention behind this is to make people smile, to lift spirits – to make a difference.

I've set a few ground rules to make it interesting and to help you (and others) get the most out of it:

1.  It must be something different each day. You can do the same thing on two different days, but it only counts the first time.

2.  You have to push yourself out of your comfort zone at least once – that is, do something that stretches you.

3.  At least one of your acts of kindness must be anonymous. That is, no one must know it was you who did it. You can't tell anyone about it.

And if you want to go even further, you can make it a 21-Day Kindness Challenge! Let me know how you get on.

# REFERENCES

## The First Side Effect: Kindness Makes Us Happier

1. S. Lyubomirsky, C. Tkach and K.M. Sheldon, 'Pursuing sustained happiness through random acts of kindness and counting one's blessings: tests of two six-week interventions', Department of Psychology, University of California, Riverside, unpublished data, 2004; *see also* https://positivepsychologyprogram.com/random-acts-kindness/

2. S.K. Nelson, K. Layous, S.W. Cole and S. Lyubomirsky, 'Do unto others or treat yourself? The effects of prosocial and self-focused behavior on psychological flourishing', *Emotion*, 21 April 2016 (advanced online publication at time of writing)

3. M.F. Steger, T.B. Kashdan and S. Oishi, 'Being good by doing good: daily eudaimonic activity and well-being', *Journal of Research in Personality* 2008, 42, 22–42

4. E.W. Dunn, L.B. Aknin and M.I. Norton, 'Spending money on others promotes happiness', *Science* 2008, 319, 1,687–8

5. L.B. Aknin, J.K. Hamlin and E.W. Dunn, 'Giving leads to happiness in young children', *PLoS ONE* 2012, 7(6), e39, 211

6. L.E. Alder and J.L. Trew, 'If it makes you happy: engaging in kind acts increases positive effect in socially anxious individuals', *Emotion* 2013, 13(1), 64–75

7.  On Patch's website, he writes, 'The Gesundheit! Institute, a non-profit healthcare organization, is a project in holistic medical care based on the belief that one cannot separate the health of the individual from the health of the family, the community, the society, and the world. Our mission is to reframe and reclaim the concept of "hospital".'

8.  Allan Luks, *The Healing Power of Doing Good*, iUniverse.com, Lincoln, NE, 1991

9.  For information on moral treatment as a historical treatment for depression, *see* T. Taubes, 'Healthy avenues of the mind: psychological theory building and the influence of religion during the era of moral treatment', *American Journal of Psychiatry* 1998, 155, 1,001–8

10. 'Mental Capital and Wellbeing: Making the most of ourselves in the 21st century', UK Government Office for Science, 2008; https://www.gov.uk/government/uploads/system/uploads/attachment_data/file/292453/mental-capital-wellbeing-summary.pdf    (last accessed 19 October 2016)

11. M.A. Musick and J. Wilson, 'Volunteering and depression: the role of psychological and social resources in different age groups', *Social Science and Medicine* 2003, 56(2), 259–69

12. E.A. Greenfield and N.F. Marks, 'Formal volunteering as a protective factor for older adults' psychological well-being', *Journal of Gerontology Series B: Psychological Sciences and Social Sciences* 2004, 59(5), S258–64

13. E. Kahana, K. Feldman, C. Fechner, E. Midlarsky and B. Kahana, 'Altruism and volunteering: effects on psychological well-being in the old-old', paper presented at the Gerontological Society of America meeting, Washington, DC, 2004

14. K.I. Hunter and M.W. Linn, 'Psychosocial differences between elderly volunteers and non-volunteers', *International Journal of Aging and Human Development* 1980–81, 12(3), 205–13

15. As recounted by Dacher Keltner. In *Born to Be Good: The Science of a Meaningful Life* (Norton, 2009), Keltner describes how

psychology professor Richie Davidson's measurement of frontal lobe activation in a Tibetan Buddhist was 'off the scale'.

16. B. Fredrickson, M. Cohn, K.A. Coffey, J. Pek and S.M. Finkel, 'Open hearts build lives: positive emotions, induced through loving-kindness meditation, build consequential personal resources', *Journal of Personality and Social Psychology* 2008, 95(5), 1,045–62

17. M. Mongrain, J.M. Chin and L.B. Shapira, 'Practicing compassion increases happiness and self-esteem', *Journal of Happiness Studies* 2011, 12, 963–81

18. R.A. Emmons and M.E. McCullough, 'Counting blessings versus burdens: an experimental investigation of gratitude and subjective well-being in daily life', *Journal of Personality and Social Psychology* 2003, 84(2), 377–89. This paper also contained the two-week study.

19. Cited in Robert A. Emmons, *Thanks: How the New Science of Gratitude Can Make You Happier*, Houghton Mifflin Harcourt, Boston, MA, 2007

## The Second Side Effect: Kindness is Good for the Heart

1. N. Magon and S. Kalra, 'The orgasmic history of oxytocin: love, lust, and labor', *Indian Journal of Endocrinology and Metabolism* 2011, 15(Suppl. 3), S156–61

2. https://en.wikipedia.org/wiki/Oxytocin

3. C. Crockford, T. Deschner, T.E. Ziegler and R.M. Wittig, 'Endogenous peripheral oxytocin measures can give insight into the dynamics of social relationships: a review', *Frontiers in Behavioural Neuroscience* 2014, 8(68), 1–14

4. M. Jankowski, T.L. Broderick and J. Gutkowska, 'Oxytocin and cardioprotection in diabetes and obesity', *BMC Endocrine Disorders* 2016, 16, 34, and M. Jankowski, A. Gonzalez-Reyes, N. Noiseux and J. Gutkowska, 'Oxytocin in the heart regeneration', *Recent Patents on Cardiovascular Drug Discovery* 2012, 7, 81–7

5.  Jankowski, Broderick and Gutkowska, ibid.

6.  F. Houshmand, M. Faghihi and S. Zahediasl, 'Role of atrial natriuretic peptide in oxytocin induced cardioprotection', *Heart, Lung and Circulation* 2015, 24(1), 86–93

7.  A. Argiolas and M.R. Melis, 'Oxytocin-induced penile erection: role of nitric oxide', *Advances in Experimental Medicine and Biology* 1995, 395, 247–54

8.  For a good video summary of nitric oxide and how it works, *see* Dr Louis Ignarro's interview: https://youtu.be/3PiljAwxS4Q

9.  Dr. Louis Ignarro and Dr Andrew Myers, *The New Heart Health*, Healthwell Ventures, Redondo Beach, CA, 2013

10. The typical responses were obtained from attendees at some of my workshops.

11. J.A. Silvers and J. Haidt, 'Moral elevation can induce nursing', *Emotion* 2008, 8(2), 291–5

12. L.J. Seltzer, T.E. Zieglar and S.D. Pollak, 'Social vocalizations can release oxytocin in humans', *Proceedings of the Royal Society B: Biological Sciences* 2010, 277(1,694), 2,661–6

13. R. White-Traut, K. Watanabe, H. Pournajafi-Nazarloo, D. Schwertz, A. Bell and C.S. Carter, 'Detection of salivary oxytocin levels in lactating women', *Developmental Psychobiology* 2009, 51(4), 367–73

14. K.M. Grewen, S.S. Girdler, J. Amico and K.C. Light, 'Effects of partner support on resting oxytocin, cortisol, norepinephrine, and blood pressure before and after warm partner contact', *Psychosomatic Medicine* 2005, 67, 531–8

15. The following review paper lists several different ways of producing oxytocin (shown in a table as well as individual discussions): C. Crockford, T. Deschner, T.E. Ziegler and R.M. Wittig, 'Endogenous peripheral oxytocin measures can give insight into the dynamics of social relationships: a review', *Frontiers in Behavioural Neuroscience* 2014, 8(68), 1–14

16. T.W. Smith, C. Berg, B.N. Uchino, P. Florsheim and G. Pearce, 'Marital conflict behavior and coronary artery calcification', Paper presented at the American Psychosomatic Society's 64th Annual

Meeting, Denver, CO, 3 March 2006, and J.K. Kiecolt-Glaser, T.J. Loving, J.R. Stowell, W.B. Malarkey, S. Lemeshow, S.L. Dickinson and R. Glaser, 'Hostile marital interactions, proinflammatory cytokine production, and wound healing', *Archives of General Psychiatry* 2005, 62, 1,377–84

17. R. Singh *et al.*, 'Role of free radical in atherosclerosis, diabetes and dyslipidaemia: larger-than-life', *Diabetes Metabolism Research and Reviews* 2015, 31(2), 113–26

18. A. Szeto, D.A. Nation, A.J. Mendez, J. Dominguez-Bendela, L.G. Brooks, N. Schneiderman and P.M. McCabe, 'Oxytocin attenuates NADP-dependent superoxide activity and IL-6 secretion in macrophages and vascular cells', *American Journal of Endrocrinology and Metabolism* 2008, 295, E1,495–1,501

19. Dr Mimi Guarneri, *The Heart Speaks*, Simon & Schuster, New York, 2006

20. Several studies are summarized in G.N. Levine, K. Allen, L.T. Braun, H.A. Christian, E. Friedmann, K.A. Taubert, S.A. Thomas, D.L. Wells, R.A. Lange, 'Pet ownership and cardiovascular risk: a scientific statement from the American Heart Association', *Circulation* 2013, 127(23), 2,353–63

21. E. Friedmann and S.A. Thomas, 'Pet ownership, social support, and one-year survival after acute myocardial infarction in the Cardiac Arrhythmia Suppression Trial (CAST)', *American Journal of Cardiology* 1995, 76, 1, 213–17

22. E. Callaway, 'Pet dogs rival humans for emotional satisfaction', *New Scientist*, 14 January 2009

23. E.B. Raposal, H.B. Laws and E.B. Ansell, 'Prosocial behavior mitigates the negative effects of stress in everyday life', *Clinical Psychological Science* 2016, 4(4), 691–8

24. Cited in Robert A. Emmons, *Thanks: How the New Science of Gratitude Can Make You Happier*, Houghton Mifflin Harcourt, Boston, MA, 2007

25. G. Affleck, H. Tennen, S. Croog and S. Levine, 'Casual attribution, perceived benefits, and morbidity after a heart attack: an 8-year

study', *Journal of Consultation and Clinical Psychology* 1987, 5(1), 29–35

26. Cited in Guarneri, op. cit.

27. K.C. Light, K.M. Grewen and J.A. Amico, 'More frequent partner hugs and higher oxytocin levels are linked to lower blood pressure and heart rate in premenopausal women', *Biological Psychology* 2005, 69, 5–21

## The Third Side Effect: Kindness Slows Ageing

1. I've done a straw poll a few times at talks. I've asked for a show of hands of who believes that their diet and lifestyle impact their health. Everyone puts their hand up. But when I've asked who believes that their rate of ageing is all in their genes, more than half (sometimes many more) put their hand up, hence I conclude that 'most' people assume...

2. C. Elabd, W. Cousin, P. Upadhyayula, R.Y. Chen, M.S. Chooljian, J. Li, S. Kung, K.P. Jiang and I.M. Conboy, 'Oxytocin is an age-specific circulating hormone that is necessary for muscle maintenance and regeneration', *Nature Communications* 2014, 5, 4,082

3. N. Gassanov, D. Devost, B. Danalache, N. Noiseux, M. Jankowski, H.H. Zingg and J. Gutkowska, 'Functional activity of the carboxyl-terminally extended oxytocin precursor peptide during cardiac differentiation of embryonic stem cells', *Stem Cells* 2008, 26, 45–54, and M. Jankowski, A. Gonzalez-Reyes, N. Noiseux and J. Gutkowska, 'Oxytocin in the heart regeneration', *Recent Patents on Cardiovascular Drug Discovery* 2012, 7, 81–7

4. For information on Polyvagal Theory, *see* https://en.wikipedia.org/wiki/Polyvagal_Theory.

5. N. Eisenberg, R.A. Fabes, P.A. Miller, J. Fultz, R. Shell, R.M. Mathy and R.R. Reno, 'Relation of sympathy and personal distress to prosocial behavior: a multimethod study', *Journal of Personality and Social Psychology* 1989, 57(1), 55–66; N. Eisenberg, M. Schaller, R.A Fabes, D. Bustamante, R.M. Mathy, R. Shell and

K. Rhodes, 'Differentiation of personal distress and sympathy in children and adults', *Developmental Psychology* 1988, 24, 766–75

6. J.E. Stellar, 'Vagal reactivity and compassionate response to the suffering of others', Dissertation submitted in partial satisfaction of the requirements for the degree of Doctor of Philosophy in Psychology, University of California at Berkeley, 2013

7. B.E. Kok, K.A. Coffey, M.A. Cohn, L.I. Catalino, T. Vacharkulksemsuk, S.B. Algoe, M. Brantley and B. Fredrickson, 'How positive emotions build physical health: perceived positive social connections account for the upward spiral between positive emotions and vagal tone', *Psychological Science* 2013, 24(7), 1,123–32

8. A good inflammaging review is C. Francheschi and J. Capisi, 'Chronic inflammation (inflammaging) and its potential contribution to age-related diseases', *Journal of Gerontology A, Biological Sciences and Medical Sciences* 2014, 69(S1), S4–S9

9. For a good review of the inflammatory reflex, *see* V.A. Pavlov and K.J. Tracey, 'The vagus nerve and the inflammatory reflex: linking immunity and metabolism', *Nature Reviews, Endocrinology* 2012, 8(12), 743–54

10. H.L. Lujan and S.E. DiCarlo, 'Physical activity, by enhancing parasympathetic tone and activating the cholinergic anti-inflammatory pathway, is a therapeutic strategy to restrain chronic inflammation and prevent many chronic diseases', *Medical Hypotheses* 2013, 80(5), 548–52. The paper suggests exercise reduces low-grade inflammation by increasing vagal tone.

11. T.W.W. Pace, L.T. Negi, D.D. Adame, S.P. Cole, T.I. Sivillia, T.D. Brown, M.J. Issa and C.L. Raison, 'Effect of compassion meditation on neuroendocrine, innate immune and behavioural responses to psychosocial stress', *Psychoneuroendocrinology* 2009, 34, 87–98. The study measured reduced inflammation in response to stress.

12. V. Deing, D. Roggenkamp, J. Kühnl, A. Gruschka, F. Stäb, H. Wenck, A. Bürkle and G. Neufang, 'Oxytocin modulates proliferation and stress responses of human skin cells: implications for atopic dermatitis', *Experimental Dermatology* 2013, 22(6), 399–405

13. For general information on nitric oxide, *see* the website of Nobel Laureate Dr Louis Ignarro: http://www.drignarro.com.

14. A.L. Sverdlov, D.T.M. Ngo, W.P.A. Chan, Y.Y. Chircov and J.D. Horowitz, 'Aging of the nitric oxide system: are we as old as our NO?', *Journal of the American Heart Association* 2014, 3, e000973

15. S.A. Austin, A.V. Santhanam and Z.S. Katusic, 'Endothelial nitric oxide modulates expression and processing of amyloid precursor protein', *Circulation Research* 2010, 107, 1,498–502. *See also* https://drnibber.com/nitric-oxide-alzheimers-disease/.

16. K.J. Kempler, D. Powell, C.C. Helms and D.B. Kin-Shapiro, 'Loving-kindness meditation's effects on nitric oxide and perceived well-being: a pilot study in experienced and inexperienced meditators', *Explore* 2015, 11(1), 32–9. The paper measures increases in nitrate and nitrite levels, which are indicative of increased nitric oxide levels.

17. I. Gusarov, L. Gautier, O. Smolentseva, I. Shamovsky, S. Eremina, A. Mironov and E. Nudler, 'Bacterial nitric oxide extends the lifespan of *C. elegans*', *Cell* 2013, 152(4), 818–30

18. G.H. Brody, T. Yu, S.R.H. Beach and R.A. Philbert, 'Prevention effects ameliorate the prospective association between nonsupportive parenting and diminished telomere length', *Prevention Science* 2015, 16(2), 171–80

19. E.A. Hoge, M.M. Chen, C.A. Metcalf, L.E. Fischer, M.H. Pollack, I. DeVivo and N.M. Simon, 'Loving-kindness meditation practice associated with longer telomeres in women', *Brain Behaviour and Immunity* 2013, 32, 159–63

20. D.C. McClelland and C. Kirshnit, 'The effect of motivational arousal through films on salivary immunoglobulin A', *Psychology and Health* 1988, 2(1), 31–52

21. G. Rein, M. Atkinson and R. McCraty, 'The physiological and psychological effects of compassion and anger', *Journal of Advancement in Medicine* 1995, 8(2), 87–105

22. D.P. Rakel, T.J. Hoeft, B.P. Barrett, B.A. Chewning, L. Marchland and M. Niu, 'Perception of empathy in the therapeutic encounter:

effects on the common cold', *Patient Education and Counselling* 2011, 85, 390–97, and D.P. Rakel, T.J. Hoeft, B.P. Barrett, B.A. Chewning, B.M. Craig and M. Niu, 'Practitioner empathy and the duration of the common cold', *Family Medicine* 2009, 41(7), 494–501

## The Fourth Side Effect: Kindness Improves Relationships

1. D.M. Buss, 'Sex differences in human mate preference: evolutionary hypothesis tested in 37 countries', *Behavioral and Brain Sciences* 1989, 12, 1–49; *see also* Dacher Keltner, *Born to Be Good: The Science of a Meaningful Life*, Norton, 2009

2. C.S. Carter, 'Oxytocin pathways and the evolution of human behaviour', *Annual Reviews in Psychology* 2014, 65, 17–39

3. https://en.wikipedia.org/wiki/Oxytocin and http://physrev.physiology.org/content/81/2/629.long

4. J. M. Gottman, *What Predicts Divorce? The Relationship between Marital Processes and Marital Outcomes*, Psychology Press, 1993. *See also* http://www.theatlantic.com/health/archive/2014/06/happily-ever-after/372573/

5. S.L. Gable, H.T. Reis, E.A. Impett and E.R. Asher, 'What do you do when things go right? The intrapersonal and interpersonal benefits of sharing positive events', *Journal of Personality and Social Psychology* 2004, 87(2), 228–45

6. Ibid.

7. S.B. Algoe, J. Haidt and S.L. Gable, 'Beyond reciprocity: gratitude and relationships in everyday life', *Emotion* 2008, 8(3), 425–9

## The Fifth Side Effect: Kindness is Contagious

1. S.B. Algoe and J. Haidt, 'Witnessing excellence in action: the other-praising emotions of elevation, gratitude, and admiration', *Journal of Positive Psychology* 2009, 4(2), 105–27

2.  J. Haidt, 'Elevation and the Positive Psychology of Morality' in C.L.M. Keys and J. Haidt (eds), *Flourishing: Positive Psychology and the Life Well-Lived*, The American Psychological Association, 2003

3.  D. Freeman, K. Aquino and B. McFerran, 'Overcoming beneficiary race as an impediment to charitable donations: social dominance orientation, the experience of moral elevation, and donation behavior', *Personality and Social Psychology Bulletin* 2009, 35, 72–94

4.  S. Schnall, J. Roper and D.M. Fessler, 'Elevation leads to altruistic behavior', *Psychological Science* 2010, 21(3), 315–20

5.  Ibid.

6.  J. Galante, M.J. Bekkers, C. Mitchell and J. Gallacher, 'Loving-kindness meditation effects on well-being and altruism: a mixed-method online RCT', *Applied Psychological Health and Wellbeing* 2016, 23 June (epub ahead of print)

7.  H. Over and M. Carpenter, 'Eighteen-month-old infants show increased helping following priming with affiliation', *Psychological Science* 2009, 20(10), 1,189–93

8.  Cited in Dacher Keltner, *Born to Be Good: The Science of a Meaningful Life*, Norton, London and New York, 2009

9.  Ibid.

10. R.A. Fabes, L.D. Hanish, C.L. Martin, A. Moss and A. Reesing, 'The effects of young children's affiliations with prosocial peers on subsequent emotionality in peer interactions', *British Journal of Developmental Psychology* 2012, 30(4), 569–85

11. R.G. Netemeyer, J.G. Maxham III, D.R. Lichenstein, 'Store manager performance and satisfaction: effects on store employee performance and satisfaction, store customer satisfaction, and store customer spending growth', *Journal of Applied Psychology* 2010, 95(3), 530–45

12. Joseph A. Chancellor, 'Ripples of generosity in the workplace: the benefits of giving, getting, and glimpsing', PhD dissertation, University of California, Riverside, December 2013

13. M. Vianello, E.M. Galliano and J. Haidt, 'Elevation at work: the effects of leaders' moral excellence', *The Journal of Positive Psychology* 2010, 5(5), 390–411

14. J.H. Fowler and N.A. Christakis, 'Dynamic spread of happiness in a large social network: longitudinal analysis over 20 years in the Framingham Heart Study', *British Medical Journal* 2008, 337, a2,338, 1–9

15. J.H. Fowler and N.A. Christakis, 'Cooperative behaviour cascades in human social networks', *Proceedings of the National Academy of Sciences* 2010, 107(12), 5,334–8

16. http://www.uwhealth.org/news/longest-kidney-chain-ever-completed-wraps-up-at-uw-hospital-and-clinics/45549 (last accessed 30 July 2016); see also http://abcnews.go.com/Health/donating-kidney-complete-stranger-order-save-loved/story?id=30288400 (last accessed 30 July 2016)

17. http://www.kidneyregistry.org

18. For information on Howard Kelly, including the 'glass of milk' account, *see* A.D. Davis, *Dr Kelly of Hopkins*, The John Hopkins Press, 1959

19. The charity my friends and I set up is Spirit Aid Foundation. The well-known actor David Hayman has been there from the very beginning and is still doing a stellar job as head of operations, dividing his time between family life, acting, filmmaking and volunteering with Spirit Aid. *See* www.spiritaid.org.

20. Ems' story comes from a Facebook page she runs called 'The Delight of Kindness'. If you want to read more stories of everyday acts of kindness, go to www.facebook.com/thedelightofkindness.

## Closing Thoughts

1. http://metro.co.uk/2016/01/26/big-issue-seller-repays-kindness-back-to-man-who-buys-him-coffee-every-week-5644613/ (last accessed 19 October 2016)

# ABOUT THE AUTHOR

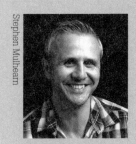

Stephen Mulhearn

**David R. Hamilton** gained a first-class honours degree in chemistry, specializing in biological and medicinal chemistry, and a PhD in organic chemistry from the University of Strathclyde in Glasgow. He holds the "slightly geeky" honour of having achieved 100% in a 3rd-year degree exam in Statistical Mechanics, a branch of quantum physics applied to chemistry.

After completing his PhD, David worked for four years in the pharmaceutical industry, developing drugs for cardiovascular disease and cancer. Upon leaving the industry, he co-founded the international relief charity Spirit Aid Foundation, and served as a director for two years.

While writing his first book, David taught chemistry, ecology and mathematics at James Watt College for Further and Higher Education, and tutored chemistry at Glasgow University. He is now the author of nine books published by Hay House, and gives talks and leads workshops that use science to inspire. David writes a regular blog on his website and occasional blogs for *Psychologies* Life Labs and *The Huffington Post.*

He has been featured in numerous publications, including *Elle*, *Red* Magazine, *Psychologies*, *YOU* Magazine, *Good Housekeeping* and several newspapers, and is also a regular contributor to BBC Radio. In 2016, David was voted Best MBS Writer by readers of *Kindred Spirit* magazine.

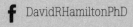 DavidRHamiltonPhD     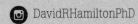 DavidRHamiltonPhD

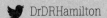 DrDRHamilton     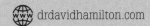 drdavidhamilton.com

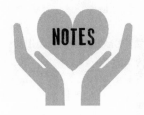

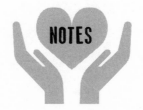

NOTES

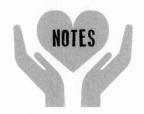

NOTES

NOTES

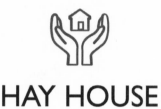

# HAY HOUSE

*Look within*

Join the conversation about latest products,
events, exclusive offers and more.

**f**  Hay House UK

🐦  @HayHouseUK

📷  @hayhouseuk

❤  healyourlife.com

*We'd love to hear from you!*